Best Me Ever!

Total Wellness Planner For Women:

D1309493

A Daily Journal and Wellness Log Book
Including
Food Diary, Fitness Journal, Meal Planner,
Weekly Planner and Daily Tracker
to Plan, Commit, and Tweak
All Areas of Your Total Wellness--
Diet, Exercise, Sleep, Mind and Spirit Health,
Social Life, Water, Steps, and Gratitude
Every Day for 91 Days/ 13 Weeks

By:
Pretty Perfect Planners

This book belongs to
the one and only:

_____

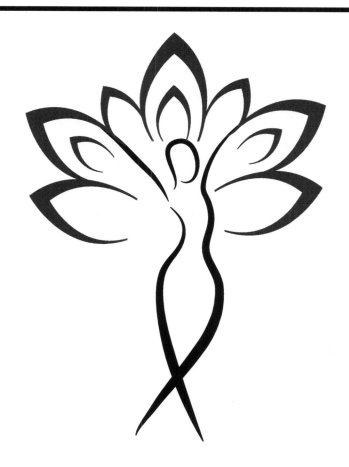

This planner/ journal was created for you! Here is your place to record your goals and track your progress as you tweak five essential health and wellness pillars in your life: diet, exercise, sleep, spirit/mind, and socialization. You've read most of the books out there on all these topics, and you know the general principles behind each one. You know about all the different diets out there (for now, at least, as more and more seem to hit the bookshelves every day). You know all about exercise, the different types you can do, the different recommendations for how much you should do, etc. You've read up on everything there is to learn about the importance of sleep hygiene and different approaches to getting your best sleep. You have heard all about the importance of spirituality, whether called mindfulness, mediation, or prayer. And finally, you know all too well that regular and meaningful social interaction is also very important to your health, and is essential to protect your brain as you age.

You've probably tried many different diets, lots of different exercise plans, and maybe even some meditation apps. Some may have worked for you, and some did not. I get it! My major pet peeve is anyone who says they have the only thing that is going to make you _____ (fill in the blank with *lose weight*, *get fit*, *reverse aging*, *prevent cancer*, *etc.*). As if we are all exactly the same, they will tell you that if you follow their diet, you will lose that excess weight, or if you follow their exercise routine, you will get fit. Regardless of what they tell you, they will conclude that their way is the only right way. If you join their social media groups, you will be banned for even asking anything about a different approach, or for suggesting that their approach is not working for you. They will tell you that you must be doing it wrong. You must be a failure.

Well--they're wrong! You are NOT a failure! You are you - - beautiful, unique, and different from anyone else who has ever been on this planet! There is no *one and only one thing* that is going to work for every body all the time. This book, however, is going to be the one thing that allows you to finally record your goals as you try some different approaches, track your progress, note what works and what doesn't work, and make small changes along the way. With this book, you will be able to tweak your health and wellness to get to the perfect plan for you -- your "best me ever!"

This book is designed to let you try the different approaches as you see fit, and record your progress, so that you can figure out what works for you! You don't fit in any one else's box! You are uniquely you, and now is the time to be the best and healthiest uniquely you you can be!

Let's go!

How To Use This Planner

   Keep in mind when using this book that each of the five essential pillars (diet, exercise, sleep, spirit/mind, and social) must be equally strong in order to hold up your total wellness. Imbalance created by weakness in even one of these pillars is going to cause the whole thing to topple!

   This journal allows you to track your progress in each of these pillars for 13 weeks, or 91 days.   Each week within this journal starts on a Monday, and ends on a Sunday. This journal is undated, although each weekday is labeled, so you can start on any Monday or other day you want, and if you skip a few days, you can resume at any later time. You will find a place to plan your weekly goals and any particular diet or other wellness approach you want to follow, or even plan just a tweak that you want to try during that time. You will also find a place to write out your weekly meal plan, and your plans for the upcoming week for exercise, mind/spirit, sleep, socialization, and even steps, water, and bedtimes. Following your weekly plan, you will find two pages for each of the upcoming days of the week. Here, you will be able to record all the details and progress as you follow your wellness plan. If you are trying intermittent fasting, there are spaces to record the opening and closing times of your eating window, as well as the total amount of time you fasted before opening your window for the day. If you are tracking carbs or fats or proteins, etc., you will find spaces to record those nutritional values, as well as others you may choose to track. This journal is designed to allow you to choose what you want to track and tweak! At the end of each week's daily records, you will find a place to reflect upon what is working and what is not. Here, you can track your biggest successes and challenges, allowing you to thoroughly evaluate your plans and consider whether to try something else.

   Sometimes, even often, a week is not enough time to see if any particular wellness habit or diet is going to work for you. Don't think that you should try a different approach each week. Instead, be patient and try something at least long enough to give it a chance. This book is all about you and you alone.   You get to go at your own pace! For example, if you want to try intermittent fasting, be aware that you may initially lose some weight very quickly, probably due to a loss of water, but then weight loss will usually slow down. You may feel anxious or grumpy at first, a feeling that usually goes away after you have fasted a few times.   It takes a while for your body to get used to a new way of eating. Give yourself to time to adjust, tweaking any given plan a bit each week, and moving on to something else after you are satisfied that you gave it enough time. Have fun on the journey! Your optimal goal will be to find that plan in each of the wellness pillars that works best for you, so that by the end of these 13 weeks, you will be much more knowledgeable about what YOUR BODY needs to be at its peak health and wellness levels.

A Few Ideas For Different Approaches You May Wish to Try

The following are some suggestions for different things you can try in each of the five total wellness pillars. This journal does not address the particulars and details of each of these plans. Instead, this book assumes that you already know what different approaches are out there, and are probably even learning more. However, below you will find a few suggestions to consider as you track and tweak your way to your best you ever!

Diet

- Vegan or Plant-based This diet includes only plant food. This includes fruit, vegetables, grains and seeds, nuts, beans and legumes. Any food that comes from animals or any living creatures (i.e., honey from bees) is excluded in this diet. The term "vegan" generally encompasses the ethical issues behind the choice to not eat food from any living thing, although the term is often used to describe people following a plant-based diet.

- Whole Food Plant Based (WFPB) This is a plant-based diet with an emphasis on only whole food, nothing processed. This means no plant-based junk food (like oreos, which are plant-based). This way of eating (WOE) focuses on whole fruits and vegetables, whole grains (intact grains, since grinding a grain is technically processing the grain), nuts, seeds, and beans. Some proponents of the WFPB WOE strictly construe the "nothing processed" component to mean also no added oil, getting oil out of any natural food involves processing. WFPB also limits anything like plant-based cheese, tofu, and any commercial plant-based meats.

- Whole Food Plant Based with No Sugar, Oil, Salt (WFPB, SOS-Free) This is the WFPB diet with an even more restrictive edge. No added sugar, oil, or salt is allowed. This WOE is based on the premise that these added ingredients are detrimental to health, and that they also artificially enhance the flavor of food, making us want to eat unnaturally more.

- Keto The Keto diet has been popular for quite a few years, but is not uncontroversial. The basic idea behind this diet is that carbohydrates must be greatly reduced to produce weight loss and greater health. The consumption of relatively high fat quantities is encouraged, while carbs are limited. Protein is maintained at a moderate level.

- Vegan Keto This twist on the Keto diet has the same tenets, yet also follows vegan diet rules, including no meat, dairy, eggs, and honey. Much of the high fat required in regular Keto diet comes from meat and dairy. With those two food groups eliminated, as well as most carbs such as grains and potatoes, the Vegan Keto diet is a very tightly defined one.

- <u>Low Carb Plant-Based</u>   Very similar to Vegan Keto, this diet focuses on a low carbohydrate consumption while eating only plant-based food, but does not look to get the body into "ketosis" in doing so. Grains, breads, pastas, rice, and potatoes are consumed in limited quantities.

- <u>High Carb Plant-Based</u>   This diet is based on the idea that carbohydrates are actually beneficial for our bodies and should be eaten in abundance to achieve total health.

- <u>Low Carb, High Fat</u>   Similar to Keto, this diet keeps carbohydrates low while allowing high fats, and is not limited to plant-based food. Therefore, dairy, meat, eggs, and cheese are big players in this diet.

- <u>Mediterranean</u>   This diet is inspired by the healthy eating habits of the lands surrounding the Mediterranean Sea. It focuses on high consumption of olive oil, legumes, fruits, whole grains, and vegetables, moderate intake of seafood, dairy, and red wine, and low intake of red meat, sweets, and carbohydrates.

- <u>Intermittent Fasting (IF)</u>   This is a WOE that cycles between periods of eating and periods of fasting. Many different variations of IF exist, predominantly 16:8 (fasting for 16 hours and eating for 8), 20:4 (fasting for 20 hours and eating for 4 hours); one meal a day (OMAD) (eating one large meal a day, and fasting the rest of the day). One keeps track of their eating window in this way of eating. When the eating window is open, one may eat, and when it is closed, there is no more eating until the next open time.

- <u>Others</u> So many other types of diets and ways of eating exist! The above list is just a small sample. The trick lies in finding the one approach, or combination of approaches that works best for you! For example, if trying IF, you may consider eating only WFPB during your eating window.

Exercise

Exercise can be done in so many different ways! What are the types of exercise that best get and keep *you* in a state of total wellness? You will find out! Here are some ideas to consider.

- Walking
- Hiking
- Swimming
- Strength training with weight or resistance bands
- Dancing
- Body weight training
- Bicycling or spinning
- High Intensity Interval Training

A complete list of different exercises to try is much too long to include here. There are also many different schools of thought as to which exercises are best for our bodies, although most do encompass both strength building as well as cardio movement. Explore different combinations to find what works best for *your* body!

Sleep

Good sleep is essential to the well-being of your body and your mind. Most experts recommend that adults get between 8-10 hours of sleep a night, and the newer focus has been on the quality of that sleep as well as the quantity. The restorative properties of sleep are enhanced when our sleep hygeine is optimum. Some things to try for ultimate sleep hygeine include the following.

- Regular bedtimes and wake times. Try not to vary your bedtimes and wake times even on the weekends.
- All electronic devices turned off at least one hour before bedtime. The blue light and other mental stimulation produced by electronic devices prevents your brain from being properly prepared for quality sleep.
- Total darkness. Even a small amount of light in the room during sleep can interfere with sleep quality.

- Cooler room temperature. Your body prefers a cool environment for best quality sleep. Experiment with different room temperatures to see what produces *your* best quality sleep.
- No food or drinks 3-4 hours before bedtime. Your digestive process interferes with sleep, and it is generally best to avoid food and drink during this time so as to promote optimal quality sleep.

Mind/Spirit

To achieve total health and wellness, you need to include a focus on the mind and spirit as well as the body. These all work together for total wellness. While a healthy body keeps you active and fit, a healthy mind and spirit keeps you focused, engaged, balanced, fulfilled, and content. Sleep, exercise, and diet all play a role in the health of your mind and spirit. However, other specific activities can greatly enhance that health. Several ideas to consider include the following.

- Mediation
- Yoga (this can actually be both a form of physical exercise and a mind exercise)
- Spending time in nature
- Prayer
- Journaling
- Engaging in hobbies
- Laughing
- Volunteering or helping others
- Reading and/or writing positive affirmations
- Taking a relaxing bath
- Practicing some self-care
- Practicing deep breathing exercises
- Writing gratitude lists
- Aromatherapy

Socialization

Social interaction is essential to every aspect of your health. Having a strong network of support and community bonds promotes both emotional and physical health. This is becoming more challenging in modern culture, with the prevalence of social media and communication through electronic devices. Face-to-face contact triggers parts of your nervous system that release neurotransmitters that help regulate your body's response to stress and anxiety. It is vital to include this component in your life to have total, balanced health and well-being. Here are just a few ideas to include as you consider how *you* want to include real social contact in your everyday life.

- Yoga class (this would be including 3 pillars in one activity--exercise, mind/spirit, and socialization)
- Meet a friend or two to go for a walk (exercise and socialization)
- Take a class, meet new people
- Girls' night out
- Meet a friend or new acquaintance for coffee or tea
- Volunteer at a local food pantry or shelter
- Stop and say hello to your neighbor
- Invite someone to join you for lunch or dinner

The ideas here are simple, and just meant to inspire you to come up with your own ideas and ways of enhancing your total wellness. You have this journal now, and now its time for you to take action! You got this!

13 WEEKS (91 DAYS) OF PROGRESS

Record your weight and/or any other parameters you want to track on the same day each week. For example, weight and steps, or sleep hours and steps, or just weight. You choose!

Starting Point	Week 1	Week 2
Week 3	Week 4	Week 5
Week 6	Week 7	Week 8
Week 9	Week 10	Week 11
Week 12	Week 13	You Did It!

My Body Measurements:

Before

Date:

After

Date:

Neck _____

Arm _____

Bust _____

Waist _____

Hips _____

Thigh _____

_____ Neck

_____ Arm

_____ Bust

_____ Waist

_____ Hips

_____ Thigh

Weight

BMI

Weight

BMI

See BMI Calculator at
cdc.gov/BMIcalculator

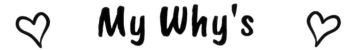

My Why's

Identifying your "why" is perhaps the most important first step in any new plan. Spend some time considering all the different reasons that motivate you to want to implement a plan to achieve total wellness. What specifically do you want to improve? How do you feel now, and how do you expect to feel when you achieve your goal? Form a vision of your future self in a state of total wellness. Return here often to remember these statements and you will find continued motivation and encouragement to persevere and keep working toward your goals. Your future self deserves this!

As I start this journal, this is how I feel about my state of wellness: _____

_____

_____

_____

_____

_____

_____

_____

_____

_____

Why I want to achieve total wellness:

_____

_____

_____

_____

_____

_____

What I intend to achieve in my diet pillar: _____

_____

_____

_____

_____

What I intend to achieve in my exercise and activity pillar: _____

_____

_____

_____

_____

_____

What I intend to achieve in my sleep habits pillar: _____

_____

_____

_____

_____

_____

What I intend to achieve in my mind/spirit pillar: _____

_____

_____

_____

_____

_____

_____

What I intend to achieve in my social life pillar: _____

_____

_____

_____

_____

_____

What are any other areas of my total health and wellness that I'd like to tweak and improve: _____

_____

_____

_____

_____

_____

What I'd like my future self to say and feel about my efforts to achieve total wellness during the next 91 days:

_____

_____

_____

_____

_____

_____

_____

_____

_____

_____

_____

You Got This!

Let's Go!

Week 1

Monday	Tuesday	Wednesday	Thursday	Friday	Saturday	Sunday
Exercise/Activity Planner						
Mind/Spirit Planner						
Social Planner						

Notes:				Bedtime Goal:	Steps Goal:	Water Goal:
				Wake-Up Goal:		

Planner

Week of: _____

Diet Goals:

Exercise Goals:

Mind Goals:

Social Goals:

Sleep Goals:

Weekly Meal Planner

Monday	Tuesday	Wednesday	Thursday	Friday	Saturday	Sunday

Weight:	# Daily

Sleep

Woke up at:	_____
Total Time Slept:	_____
Tonight's Bedtime:	_____
Time Electronics Off:	_____
Time Lights Off:	_____
Room Temperature:	_____
Notes:	_____

Mind /Spirit

What I did:	Time Spent:

Social

Activity:	Time Spent:

Gratitude / Reflections

Record

Date: Monday / /

Food

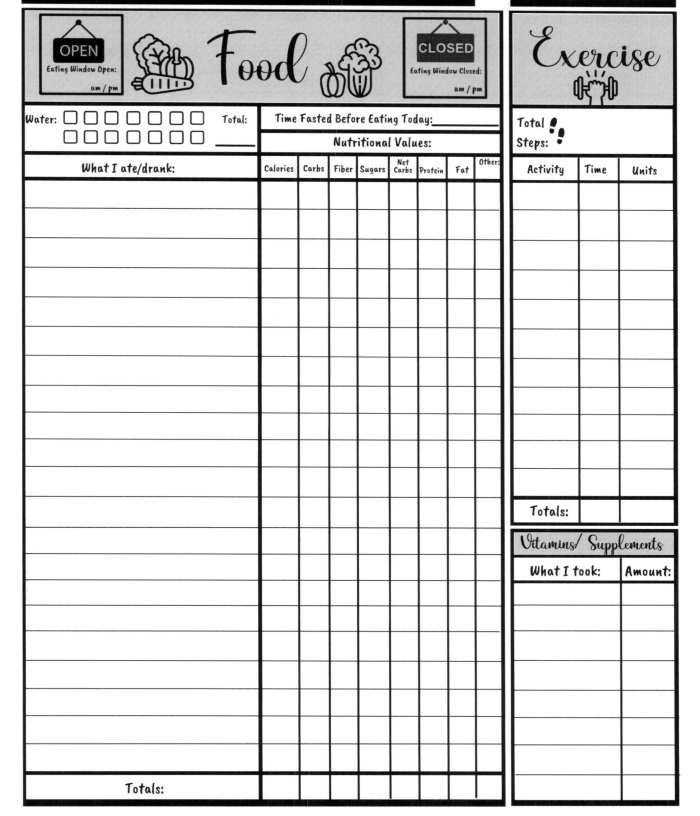

OPEN Eating Window Open: ___ am / pm

CLOSED Eating Window Closed: ___ am / pm

Water: ☐☐☐☐☐☐☐ ☐☐☐☐☐☐☐ Total: ____

Time Fasted Before Eating Today: _____

Nutritional Values:

What I ate/drank:	Calories	Carbs	Fiber	Sugars	Net Carbs	Protein	Fat	Other:
Totals:								

Exercise

Total Steps:

Activity	Time	Units
Totals:		

Vitamins/ Supplements

What I took:	Amount:

Weight:	# Daily

Sleep

Woke up at: _____

Total Time Slept: _____

Tonight's Bedtime: _____

Time Electronics Off: _____

Time Lights Off: _____

Room Temperature: _____

Notes: _____

_____

_____

_____

Mind / Spirit

What I did:	Time Spent:

Social

Activity:	Time Spent:

♡ Gratitude / Reflections ♡

Record

Food

OPEN
Eating Window Open:
am / pm

CLOSED
Eating Window Closed:
am / pm

Exercise

Water: ☐ ☐ ☐ ☐ ☐ ☐ ☐   Total: _____
☐ ☐ ☐ ☐ ☐ ☐ _____

Time Fasted Before Eating Today: _____

Nutritional Values:

Total Steps:

What I ate/drank:	Calories	Carbs	Fiber	Sugars	Net Carbs	Protein	Fat	Other:
Totals:								

Activity	Time	Units
Totals:		

Vitamins/ Supplements

What I took:	Amount:

Weight:	# Daily

Sleep

Woke up at: _____

Total Time Slept: _____

Tonight's Bedtime: _____

Time Electronics Off: _____

Time Lights Off: _____

Room Temperature: _____

Notes: _____

_____

_____

_____

Mind / Spirit

What I did:	Time Spent:

Social

Activity:	Time Spent:

Gratitude / Reflections

Record

Food

OPEN
Eating Window Open:
___ am / pm

CLOSED
Eating Window Closed:
___ am / pm

Exercise

Water: ☐ ☐ ☐ ☐ ☐ ☐ Total:
☐ ☐ ☐ ☐ ☐ ☐ ___

Time Fasted Before Eating Today: _____

Nutritional Values:

Total Steps:

What I ate/drank:	Calories	Carbs	Fiber	Sugars	Net Carbs	Protein	Fat	Other:
Totals:								

Activity	Time	Units
Totals:		

Vitamins/ Supplements

What I took:	Amount:

Daily

Sleep

Woke up at: _____

Total Time Slept: _____

Tonight's Bedtime: _____

Time Electronics Off: _____

Time Lights Off: _____

Room Temperature: _____

Notes: _____

_____

_____

_____

Mind /Spirit

What I did:	Time Spent:

Social

Activity:	Time Spent:

Gratitude / Reflections

Weight: _____

Record

Food

OPEN
Eating Window Open:
am / pm

CLOSED
Eating Window Closed:
am / pm

Exercise

Water: ☐☐☐☐☐☐ Total: ☐☐☐☐☐☐ _____

Time Fasted Before Eating Today: _____

Nutritional Values:

Total Steps:

What I ate/drank:	Calories	Carbs	Fiber	Sugars	Net Carbs	Protein	Fat	Other:
Totals:								

Activity	Time	Units
Totals:		

Vitamins/ Supplements

What I took:	Amount:

Weight:	**Daily**

Sleep

Woke up at: _____

Total Time Slept: _____

Tonight's Bedtime: _____

Time Electronics Off: _____

Time Lights Off: _____

Room Temperature: _____

Notes: _____

_____

_____

_____

Mind / Spirit

What I did:	Time Spent:

Social

Activity:	Time Spent:

Gratitude / Reflections

Record

Food

OPEN — Eating Window Open: ___ am / pm

CLOSED — Eating Window Closed: ___ am / pm

Exercise

Water: ☐☐☐☐☐☐☐ ☐☐☐☐☐☐☐ Total: _____

Time Fasted Before Eating Today: _____

Nutritional Values:

Total Steps:

What I ate/drank:	Calories	Carbs	Fiber	Sugars	Net Carbs	Protein	Fat	Other:
Totals:								

Activity	Time	Units
Totals:		

Vitamins/ Supplements

What I took:	Amount:

Weight:	# Daily

Sleep

Woke up at: _____

Total Time Slept: _____

Tonight's Bedtime: _____

Time Electronics Off: _____

Time Lights Off: _____

Room Temperature: _____

Notes: _____

_____

_____

_____

Mind / Spirit

What I did:	Time Spent:

Social

Activity:	Time Spent:

Gratitude / Reflections

Record

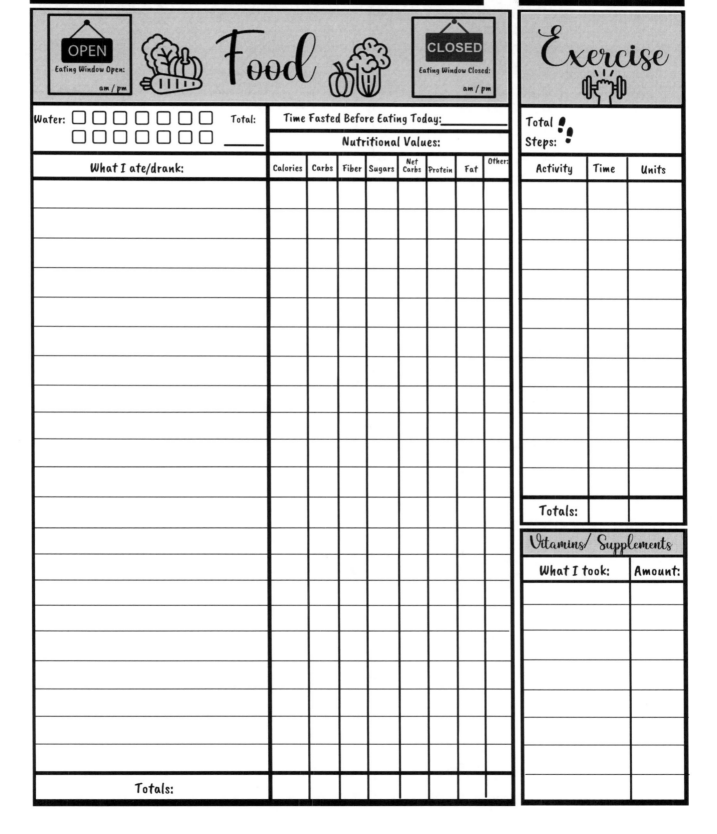

Date: Saturday / /

Food

OPEN — Eating Window Open: ___ am / pm

CLOSED — Eating Window Closed: ___ am / pm

Exercise

Water: ☐☐☐☐☐☐ ☐☐☐☐☐☐ Total: ____

Time Fasted Before Eating Today: _____

Nutritional Values:

What I ate/drank:	Calories	Carbs	Fiber	Sugars	Net Carbs	Protein	Fat	Other:
Totals:								

Total Steps:

Activity	Time	Units
Totals:		

Vitamins/ Supplements

What I took:	Amount:

Daily

Sleep

Woke up at: _____

Total Time Slept: _____

Tonight's Bedtime: _____

Time Electronics Off: _____

Time Lights Off: _____

Room Temperature: _____

Notes: _____

_____

_____

_____

Mind /Spirit

What I did:	Time Spent:

Social

Activity:	Time Spent:

Gratitude / Reflections

Weight: _____

Record

Food

OPEN
Eating Window Open:
_____ am / pm

CLOSED
Eating Window Closed:
_____ am / pm

Exercise

Water: ☐☐☐☐☐☐☐ Total: _____
☐☐☐☐☐☐☐

Time Fasted Before Eating Today: _____

Nutritional Values:

Total Steps:

What I ate/drank:	Calories	Carbs	Fiber	Sugars	Net Carbs	Protein	Fat	Other:
Totals:								

Activity	Time	Units
Totals:		

Vitamins/ Supplements

What I took:	Amount:

Weight Change:

Review

Sleep

Average Sleep Time: _____

What worked: _____

_____

What I can improve: _____

_____

Any changes I'd like to try next week: _____

_____

_____

_____

Mind /Spirit

What worked: _____

_____

What I can improve: _____

_____

Any changes I'd like to try next week:_____

_____

_____

_____

Social

What I enjoyed the most:_____

_____

_____

What I can improve next week:_____

_____

_____

_____

Ideas for other social interaction next week:_____

_____

_____

_____

♡ Gratitude / Reflections ♡

What I am grateful for as I review this week:_____

_____

_____

_____

_____

Positive reflections to carry into next week:_____

_____

_____

_____

_____

Last Week

Food

Daily average amount of water: _____

What worked: _____
_____

What I can improve: _____
_____

How I did with calories/nutrients measured: _____
_____

How I can improve: _____
_____
_____

How I did with other diet goals: _____

How I can improve: _____
_____
_____

Overall how I felt about what I consumed this week: _____

What I'd like to improve next week: _____

Exercise

Average
Daily Steps: _____

What I enjoyed most: _____

What I can improve: _____

Vitamins/ Supplements

Any impact I noticed: _____

Any changes to try: _____

Week 2

Monday	Tuesday	Wednesday	Thursday	Friday	Saturday	Sunday
Exercise/Activity Planner						
Mind/Spirit Planner						
Social Planner						

Notes:

Bedtime Goal:

Wake-Up Goal:

Steps Goal:

Water Goal:

Planner

Week of: _____

Diet Goals:

Exercise Goals:

Mind Goals:

Social Goals:

Sleep Goals:

Weekly Meal Planner

Monday	Tuesday	Wednesday	Thursday	Friday	Saturday	Sunday

Daily

Weight:

Sleep

Woke up at: _____

Total Time Slept: _____

Tonight's Bedtime: _____

Time Electronics Off: _____

Time Lights Off: _____

Room Temperature: _____

Notes: _____

_____

_____

_____

Mind / Spirit

What I did:	Time Spent:

Social

Activity:	Time Spent:

Gratitude / Reflections

Record

Food

OPEN — Eating Window Open: ___ am / pm

CLOSED — Eating Window Closed: ___ am / pm

Water: ☐☐☐☐☐☐ ☐☐☐☐☐☐ Total: ___

Time Fasted Before Eating Today: _____

Nutritional Values:

What I ate/drank:	Calories	Carbs	Fiber	Sugars	Net Carbs	Protein	Fat	Other:
Totals:								

Exercise

Total Steps: ___

Activity	Time	Units
Totals:		

Vitamins/ Supplements

What I took:	Amount:

Weight:

Daily

Sleep

Woke up at:	
Total Time Slept:	
Tonight's Bedtime:	
Time Electronics Off:	
Time Lights Off:	
Room Temperature:	
Notes:	

Mind / Spirit

What I did:	Time Spent:

Social

Activity:	Time Spent:

Gratitude / Reflections

Record

Date: Tuesday / /

Food

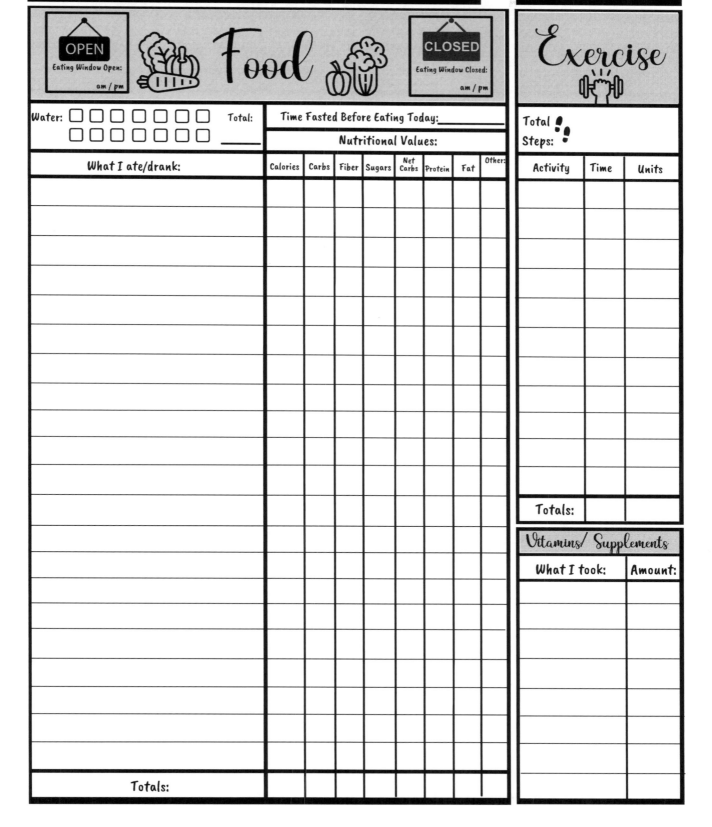

OPEN — Eating Window Open: ___ am / pm

CLOSED — Eating Window Closed: ___ am / pm

Water: ☐☐☐☐☐☐ ☐☐☐☐☐☐ Total: _____

Time Fasted Before Eating Today: _____

Nutritional Values:

What I ate/drank:	Calories	Carbs	Fiber	Sugars	Net Carbs	Protein	Fat	Other:
Totals:								

Exercise

Total Steps:

Activity	Time	Units
Totals:		

Vitamins/ Supplements

What I took:	Amount:

Weight:		**Daily**

Sleep

Woke up at:	_____
Total Time Slept:	_____
Tonight's Bedtime:	_____
Time Electronics Off:	_____
Time Lights Off:	_____
Room Temperature:	_____
Notes:	_____

Mind / Spirit

What I did:	Time Spent:

Social

Activity:	Time Spent:

Gratitude / Reflections

Record

Food

OPEN
Eating Window Open:
am / pm

CLOSED
Eating Window Closed:
am / pm

Exercise

Water: ☐ ☐ ☐ ☐ ☐ ☐ ☐   Total: ____
☐ ☐ ☐ ☐ ☐ ☐

Time Fasted Before Eating Today: _____

Nutritional Values:

Total Steps:

What I ate/drank:	Calories	Carbs	Fiber	Sugars	Net Carbs	Protein	Fat	Other:
Totals:								

Activity	Time	Units
Totals:		

Vitamins/ Supplements

What I took:	Amount:

Weight:	# Daily

Sleep

Woke up at: _____

Total Time Slept: _____

Tonight's Bedtime: _____

Time Electronics Off: _____

Time Lights Off: _____

Room Temperature: _____

Notes: _____

_____

_____

_____

Mind / Spirit

What I did:	Time Spent:

Social

Activity:	Time Spent:

Gratitude / Reflections

Record

Food

OPEN Eating Window Open: ___ am / pm

CLOSED Eating Window Closed: ___ am / pm

Exercise

Water: ☐☐☐☐☐☐☐ Total: _____
☐☐☐☐☐☐☐

Time Fasted Before Eating Today: _____

Nutritional Values:

What I ate/drank:	Calories	Carbs	Fiber	Sugars	Net Carbs	Protein	Fat	Other:
Totals:								

Total Steps:

Activity	Time	Units
Totals:		

Vitamins/ Supplements

What I took:	Amount:

Weight:	# Daily

Sleep

Woke up at: _____

Total Time Slept: _____

Tonight's Bedtime: _____

Time Electronics Off: _____

Time Lights Off: _____

Room Temperature: _____

Notes: _____

_____

_____

_____

Mind / Spirit

What I did:	Time Spent:

Social

Activity:	Time Spent:

Gratitude / Reflections

Record

Food

OPEN — Eating Window Open: ___ am / pm

CLOSED — Eating Window Closed: ___ am / pm

Exercise

Water: ☐☐☐☐☐☐☐ ☐☐☐☐☐☐ Total: ____

Time Fasted Before Eating Today: _____

Nutritional Values:

Total Steps:

What I ate/drank:	Calories	Carbs	Fiber	Sugars	Net Carbs	Protein	Fat	Other:
Totals:								

Activity	Time	Units
Totals:		

Vitamins/ Supplements

What I took:	Amount:

Weight:	**Daily**

Sleep

Woke up at: _____

Total Time Slept: _____

Tonight's Bedtime: _____

Time Electronics Off: _____

Time Lights Off: _____

Room Temperature: _____

Notes: _____

Mind / Spirit

What I did:	Time Spent:

Social

Activity:	Time Spent:

Gratitude / Reflections

Record

Food

OPEN — Eating Window Open: ___ am / pm

CLOSED — Eating Window Closed: ___ am / pm

Exercise

Water: ☐☐☐☐☐☐ ☐☐☐☐☐☐   Total: ____

Time Fasted Before Eating Today: _____

Nutritional Values:

Total Steps:

What I ate/drank:	Calories	Carbs	Fiber	Sugars	Net Carbs	Protein	Fat	Other:
Totals:								

Activity	Time	Units
Totals:		

Vitamins/ Supplements

What I took:	Amount:

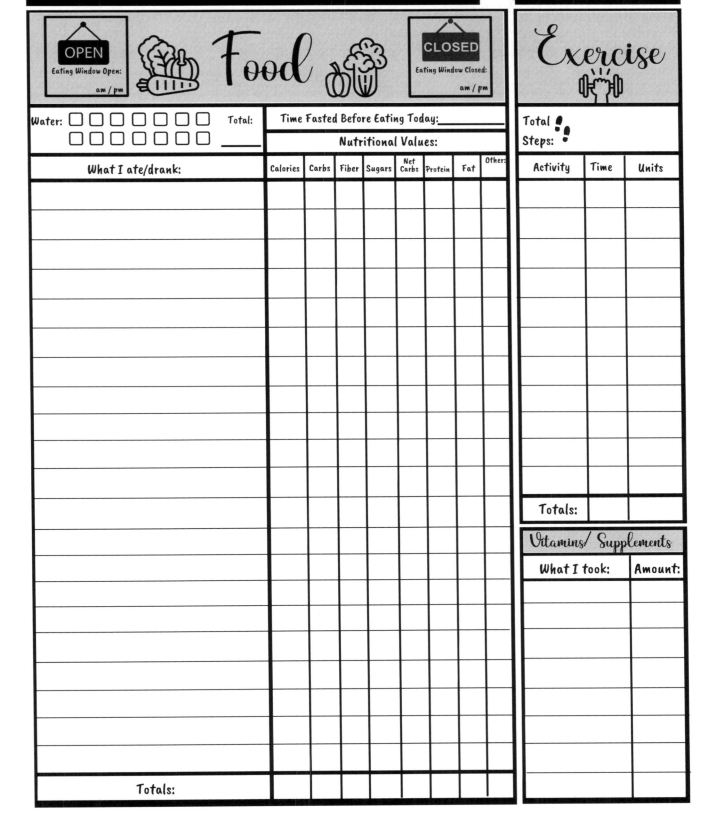

Weight:

Daily

Sleep

Woke up at: _____

Total Time Slept: _____

Tonight's Bedtime: _____

Time Electronics Off: _____

Time Lights Off: _____

Room Temperature: _____

Notes: _____

_____

_____

_____

Mind / Spirit

What I did:	Time Spent:

Social

Activity:	Time Spent:

Gratitude / Reflections

Record

Food

OPEN Eating Window Open: ___ am / pm

CLOSED Eating Window Closed: ___ am / pm

Exercise

Water: ☐☐☐☐☐☐☐ ☐☐☐☐☐☐☐ Total: ___

Time Fasted Before Eating Today: _____

Nutritional Values:

Total Steps:

What I ate/drank:	Calories	Carbs	Fiber	Sugars	Net Carbs	Protein	Fat	Other:
Totals:								

Activity	Time	Units
Totals:		

Vitamins/ Supplements

What I took:	Amount:

Weight Change:	# Review

Sleep

Average Sleep Time: _____

What worked: _____

What I can improve: _____
_____

Any changes I'd like to try next week: _____
_____
_____
_____

Mind / Spirit

What worked: _____
_____

What I can improve: _____
_____

Any changes I'd like to try next week: _____
_____
_____
_____

Social

What I enjoyed the most: _____
_____

What I can improve next week: _____
_____
_____

Ideas for other social interaction next week: _____
_____
_____
_____
_____

♡ Gratitude / Reflections ♡

What I am grateful for as I review this week: _____
_____
_____
_____
_____

Positive reflections to carry into next week: _____
_____
_____
_____

Last Week

Food

Daily average amount of water: _____

    What worked: _____
_____

    What I can improve: _____
_____

How I did with calories/nutrients measured: _____
_____

    How I can improve: _____
_____
_____

How I did with other diet goals: _____
_____

    How I can improve: _____
_____
_____

Overall how I felt about what I consumed this week: _____
_____

What I'd like to improve next week: _____
_____

Exercise

Average
Daily Steps: _____

What I enjoyed most: _____
_____
_____
_____

What I can improve: _____
_____
_____
_____
_____
_____

Vitamins/ Supplements

Any impact I noticed: _____
_____
_____

Any changes to try: _____
_____
_____
_____

Week 3

Monday	Tuesday	Wednesday	Thursday	Friday	Saturday	Sunday
Exercise/Activity Planner						
Mind/Spirit Planner						
Social Planner						

Notes:			Bedtime Goal:	Steps Goal:	Water Goal:
			Wake-Up Goal:		

Planner

Diet Goals:

Exercise Goals:

Mind Goals:

Social Goals:

Sleep Goals:

Weekly Meal Planner

Monday	Tuesday	Wednesday	Thursday	Friday	Saturday	Sunday

Weight:	# Daily

Sleep

Woke up at: _____

Total Time Slept: _____

Tonight's Bedtime: _____

Time Electronics Off: _____

Time Lights Off: _____

Room Temperature: _____

Notes: _____

_____

_____

_____

Mind / Spirit

What I did:	Time Spent:

Social

Activity:	Time Spent:

Gratitude / Reflections

Record

Food

OPEN — Eating Window Open: ___ am / pm

CLOSED — Eating Window Closed: ___ am / pm

Exercise

Water: ☐☐☐☐☐☐☐ ☐☐☐☐☐☐ Total: _____

Time Fasted Before Eating Today: _____

Nutritional Values:

Total Steps:

What I ate/drank:	Calories	Carbs	Fiber	Sugars	Net Carbs	Protein	Fat	Other:
Totals:								

Activity	Time	Units
Totals:		

Vitamins/ Supplements

What I took:	Amount:

Weight:	# Daily

Sleep

Woke up at: _____

Total Time Slept: _____

Tonight's Bedtime: _____

Time Electronics Off: _____

Time Lights Off: _____

Room Temperature: _____

Notes: _____

_____

_____

_____

Mind / Spirit

What I did:	Time Spent:

Social

Activity:	Time Spent:

♡ Gratitude / Reflections ♡

_____

_____

_____

_____

_____

_____

_____

_____

_____

_____

_____

Record

Food

OPEN Eating Window Open: ___ am / pm

CLOSED Eating Window Closed: ___ am / pm

Exercise

Water: ☐ ☐ ☐ ☐ ☐ ☐ ☐   Total: ____
☐ ☐ ☐ ☐ ☐ ☐

Time Fasted Before Eating Today: _____

Nutritional Values:

Total Steps:

What I ate/drank:	Calories	Carbs	Fiber	Sugars	Net Carbs	Protein	Fat	Other:
Totals:								

Activity	Time	Units
Totals:		

Vitamins/ Supplements

What I took:	Amount:

Weight:	# Daily

Sleep

Woke up at:	
Total Time Slept:	
Tonight's Bedtime:	
Time Electronics Off:	
Time Lights Off:	
Room Temperature:	
Notes:	

Mind / Spirit

What I did:	Time Spent:

Social

Activity:	Time Spent:

Gratitude / Reflections

Record

Food

OPEN — Eating Window Open: ___ am / pm

CLOSED — Eating Window Closed: ___ am / pm

Exercise

Water: ☐ ☐ ☐ ☐ ☐ ☐ ☐
☐ ☐ ☐ ☐ ☐ ☐
Total: _____

Time Fasted Before Eating Today: _____

Nutritional Values:

Total Steps:

What I ate/drank:	Calories	Carbs	Fiber	Sugars	Net Carbs	Protein	Fat	Other:
Totals:								

Activity	Time	Units
Totals:		

Vitamins/ Supplements

What I took:	Amount:

| Weight: | **Daily** |

Sleep

Woke up at:	_____
Total Time Slept:	_____
Tonight's Bedtime:	_____
Time Electronics Off:	_____
Time Lights Off:	_____
Room Temperature:	_____
Notes:	_____

Mind / Spirit

What I did:	Time Spent:

Social

Activity:	Time Spent:

Gratitude / Reflections

Record

Food

OPEN — Eating Window Open: __ am / pm

CLOSED — Eating Window Closed: __ am / pm

Exercise

Water: ☐ ☐ ☐ ☐ ☐ ☐ ☐ ☐ ☐ ☐ ☐ ☐ ☐ ☐   Total: _____

Time Fasted Before Eating Today: _____

Nutritional Values:

Total Steps:

What I ate/drank:	Calories	Carbs	Fiber	Sugars	Net Carbs	Protein	Fat	Other:
Totals:								

Activity	Time	Units
Totals:		

Vitamins/ Supplements

What I took:	Amount:

Weight:	# Daily

Sleep

Woke up at: _____

Total Time Slept: _____

Tonight's Bedtime: _____

Time Electronics Off: _____

Time Lights Off: _____

Room Temperature: _____

Notes: _____

_____

_____

_____

Mind / Spirit

What I did:	Time Spent:

Social

Activity:	Time Spent:

Gratitude / Reflections

Record

Date: Friday / /

Food

OPEN
Eating Window Open:
____ am / pm

CLOSED
Eating Window Closed:
____ am / pm

Exercise

Water: ☐ ☐ ☐ ☐ ☐ ☐ ☐ ☐ ☐ ☐ ☐ ☐ Total: ____

Time Fasted Before Eating Today: ____

Nutritional Values:

Total Steps:

What I ate/drank:	Calories	Carbs	Fiber	Sugars	Net Carbs	Protein	Fat	Other:
Totals:								

Activity	Time	Units
Totals:		

Vitamins/ Supplements

What I took:	Amount:

Weight:	

Daily

Sleep

Woke up at: _____

Total Time Slept: _____

Tonight's Bedtime: _____

Time Electronics Off: _____

Time Lights Off: _____

Room Temperature: _____

Notes: _____

_____

_____

_____

Mind / Spirit

What I did:	Time Spent:

Social

Activity:	Time Spent:

Gratitude / Reflections

Record

Food

OPEN Eating Window Open: ___ am / pm

CLOSED Eating Window Closed: ___ am / pm

Exercise

Water: ☐ ☐ ☐ ☐ ☐ ☐ ☐
☐ ☐ ☐ ☐ ☐ ☐

Total: _____

Time Fasted Before Eating Today: _____

Nutritional Values:

Total Steps:

What I ate/drank:	Calories	Carbs	Fiber	Sugars	Net Carbs	Protein	Fat	Other:
Totals:								

Activity	Time	Units
Totals:		

Vitamins/ Supplements

What I took:	Amount:

	Weight:		# Daily

Sleep

Woke up at: _____

Total Time Slept: _____

Tonight's Bedtime: _____

Time Electronics Off: _____

Time Lights Off: _____

Room Temperature: _____

Notes: _____

_____

_____

_____

Mind / Spirit

What I did:	Time Spent:

Social

Activity:	Time Spent:

♡ Gratitude / Reflections ♡

Record

Food

OPEN Eating Window Open: ___ am / pm

CLOSED Eating Window Closed: ___ am / pm

Exercise

Water: ☐☐☐☐☐☐ ☐☐☐☐☐☐ Total: ____

Time Fasted Before Eating Today: _____

Nutritional Values:

Total Steps:

What I ate/drank:	Calories	Carbs	Fiber	Sugars	Net Carbs	Protein	Fat	Other:
Totals:								

Activity	Time	Units
Totals:		

Vitamins/ Supplements

What I took:	Amount:

Weight Change:	# Review

Sleep

Average Sleep Time: _____

What worked: _____

_____

What I can improve: _____

_____

_____

Any changes I'd like to try next week: _____

_____

_____

_____

Mind / Spirit

What worked: _____

_____

What I can improve: _____

_____

_____

Any changes I'd like to try next week: _____

_____

_____

_____

Social

What I enjoyed the most: _____

_____

_____

What I can improve next week: _____

_____

_____

_____

Ideas for other social interaction next week: _____

_____

_____

_____

_____

♡ Gratitude / Reflections ♡

What I am grateful for as I review this week: _____

_____

_____

_____

_____

Positive reflections to carry into next week: _____

_____

_____

_____

Last Week

Food

Daily average amount of water: _____

What worked: _____
_____

What I can improve: _____
_____

How I did with calories/nutrients measured: _____
_____

How I can improve: _____
_____
_____

How I did with other diet goals: _____
_____

How I can improve: _____
_____
_____

Overall how I felt about what I consumed this week: _____
_____

What I'd like to improve next week: _____
_____
_____

Exercise

Average Daily Steps: _____

What I enjoyed most: _____

What I can improve: _____

Vitamins/ Supplements

Any impact I noticed: _____

Any changes to try: _____

Week 4

Weekly

Monday	Tuesday	Wednesday	Thursday	Friday	Saturday	Sunday
Exercise/Activity Planner						
Mind/Spirit Planner						
Social Planner						

Notes:

Bedtime Goal:

Wake-Up Goal:

Steps Goal:

Water Goal:

Planner

Week of: _____

Diet Goals:

Exercise Goals:

Mind Goals:

Social Goals:

Sleep Goals:

Weekly Meal Planner

Monday	Tuesday	Wednesday	Thursday	Friday	Saturday	Sunday

Weight:	# Daily

Sleep

Woke up at: _____

Total Time Slept: _____

Tonight's Bedtime: _____

Time Electronics Off: _____

Time Lights Off: _____

Room Temperature: _____

Notes: _____

_____

_____

_____

Mind /Spirit

What I did:	Time Spent:

Social

Activity:	Time Spent:

Gratitude / Reflections

Record

Date: Monday / /

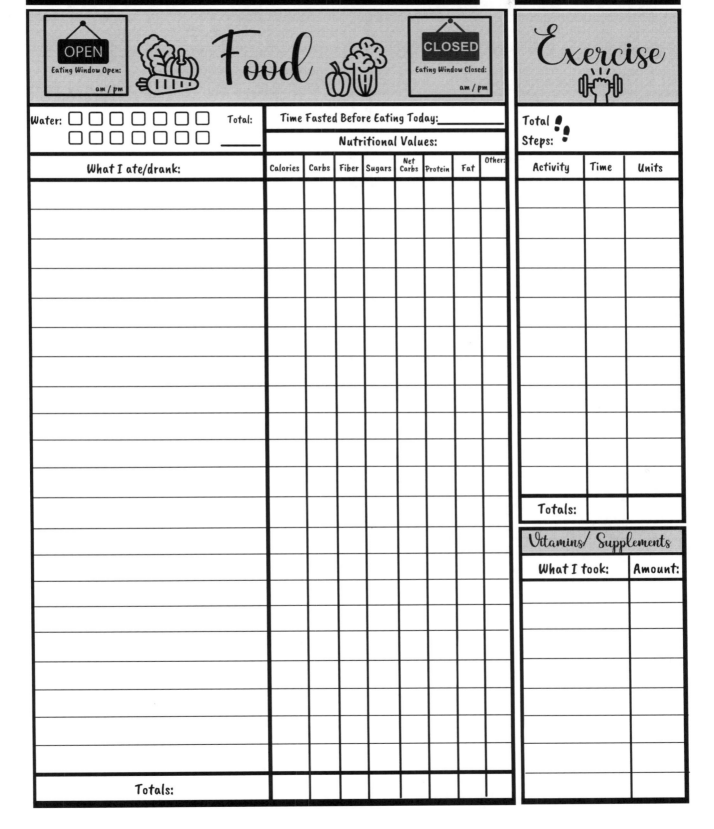

Food

OPEN — Eating Window Open: ___ am / pm

CLOSED — Eating Window Closed: ___ am / pm

Exercise

Water: ☐☐☐☐☐☐ ☐☐☐☐☐☐ Total: _____

Time Fasted Before Eating Today: _____

Nutritional Values:

Total Steps:

What I ate/drank:	Calories	Carbs	Fiber	Sugars	Net Carbs	Protein	Fat	Other:
Totals:								

Activity	Time	Units
Totals:		

Vitamins/ Supplements

What I took:	Amount:

Weight:	**Daily**

Sleep

Woke up at: _____

Total Time Slept: _____

Tonight's Bedtime: _____

Time Electronics Off: _____

Time Lights Off: _____

Room Temperature: _____

Notes: _____

_____

_____

_____

Mind / Spirit

What I did:	Time Spent:

Social

Activity:	Time Spent:

Gratitude / Reflections

Record

Food

OPEN — Eating Window Open: _____ am / pm

CLOSED — Eating Window Closed: _____ am / pm

Exercise

Water: ☐☐☐☐☐☐☐ ☐☐☐☐☐☐ Total: _____

Time Fasted Before Eating Today: _____

Nutritional Values:

Total Steps:

What I ate/drank:	Calories	Carbs	Fiber	Sugars	Net Carbs	Protein	Fat	Other:
Totals:								

Activity	Time	Units
Totals:		

Vitamins/ Supplements

What I took:	Amount:

Weight:	

Daily

Sleep

Woke up at:	
Total Time Slept:	
Tonight's Bedtime:	
Time Electronics Off:	
Time Lights Off:	
Room Temperature:	
Notes:	

Mind / Spirit

What I did:	Time Spent:

Social

Activity:	Time Spent:

Gratitude / Reflections

Record

Food

OPEN
Eating Window Open:
am / pm

CLOSED
Eating Window Closed:
am / pm

Exercise

Water: ☐ ☐ ☐ ☐ ☐ ☐ ☐   Total: _____
☐ ☐ ☐ ☐ ☐ ☐ ☐

Time Fasted Before Eating Today: _____

Total Steps:

Nutritional Values:

What I ate/drank:	Calories	Carbs	Fiber	Sugars	Net Carbs	Protein	Fat	Other:
Totals:								

Activity	Time	Units
Totals:		

Vitamins/ Supplements

What I took:	Amount:

Weight:	

Daily

Sleep

Woke up at: _____

Total Time Slept: _____

Tonight's Bedtime: _____

Time Electronics Off: _____

Time Lights Off: _____

Room Temperature: _____

Notes: _____

_____

_____

_____

Mind / Spirit

What I did:	Time Spent:

Social

Activity:	Time Spent:

Gratitude / Reflections

Record

Food

OPEN — Eating Window Open: ___ am / pm

CLOSED — Eating Window Closed: ___ am / pm

Exercise

Water: ☐☐☐☐☐☐☐ ☐☐☐☐☐☐ Total: ____

Time Fasted Before Eating Today: _____

Total Steps:

Nutritional Values:

What I ate/drank:	Calories	Carbs	Fiber	Sugars	Net Carbs	Protein	Fat	Other:
Totals:								

Activity	Time	Units
Totals:		

Vitamins/ Supplements

What I took:	Amount:

Weight:	# Daily

Sleep

Woke up at: _____

Total Time Slept: _____

Tonight's Bedtime: _____

Time Electronics Off: _____

Time Lights Off: _____

Room Temperature: _____

Notes: _____

_____

_____

_____

Mind / Spirit

What I did:	Time Spent:

Social

Activity:	Time Spent:

Gratitude / Reflections

Record

Food

OPEN Eating Window Open: ___ am / pm

CLOSED Eating Window Closed: ___ am / pm

Exercise

Water: ☐☐☐☐☐☐☐ ☐☐☐☐☐☐☐   Total: _____

Time Fasted Before Eating Today: _____

Nutritional Values:

What I ate/drank:	Calories	Carbs	Fiber	Sugars	Net Carbs	Protein	Fat	Other:
Totals:								

Total Steps:

Activity	Time	Units
Totals:		

Vitamins/ Supplements

What I took:	Amount:

Weight:	# Daily

Sleep

Woke up at: _____

Total Time Slept: _____

Tonight's Bedtime: _____

Time Electronics Off: _____

Time Lights Off: _____

Room Temperature: _____

Notes: _____

_____

_____

_____

Mind / Spirit

What I did:	Time Spent:

Social

Activity:	Time Spent:

Gratitude / Reflections

Record

Date: Saturday ___/___/___

Food

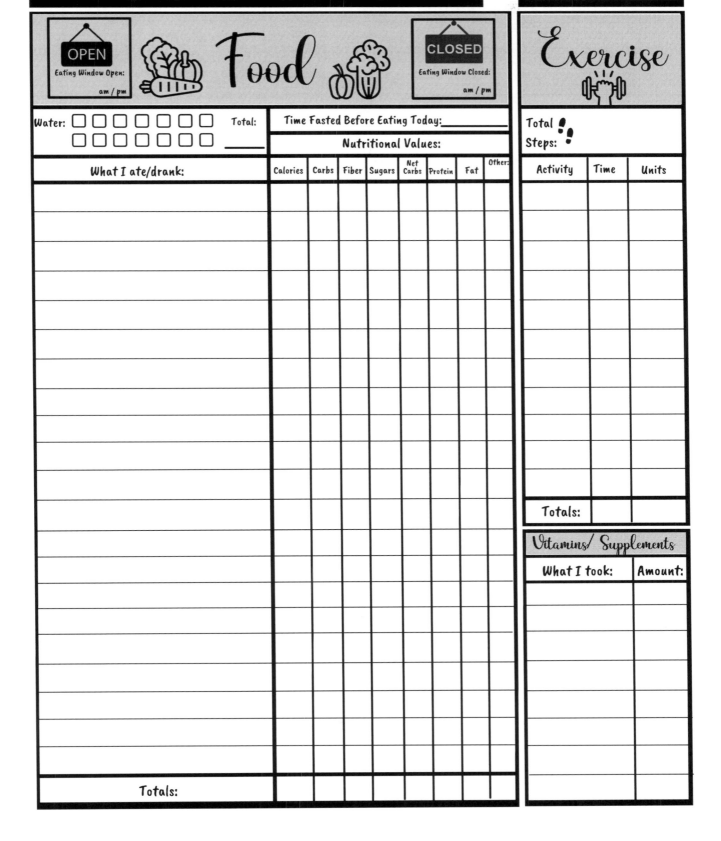

OPEN — Eating Window Open: ___ am / pm

CLOSED — Eating Window Closed: ___ am / pm

Water: ☐☐☐☐☐☐☐ ☐☐☐☐☐☐ Total: _____

Time Fasted Before Eating Today: _____

Nutritional Values:

What I ate/drank:	Calories	Carbs	Fiber	Sugars	Net Carbs	Protein	Fat	Other:
Totals:								

Exercise

Total Steps: _____

Activity	Time	Units
Totals:		

Vitamins/ Supplements

What I took:	Amount:

Daily

Weight:

Sleep

Woke up at: _____

Total Time Slept: _____

Tonight's Bedtime: _____

Time Electronics Off: _____

Time Lights Off: _____

Room Temperature: _____

Notes: _____

_____

_____

_____

Mind / Spirit

What I did:	Time Spent:

Social

Activity:	Time Spent:

♡ Gratitude / Reflections ♡

Record

Food

OPEN Eating Window Open: ___ am / pm

CLOSED Eating Window Closed: ___ am / pm

Exercise

Water: ☐ ☐ ☐ ☐ ☐ ☐ ☐   Total: ___
☐ ☐ ☐ ☐ ☐ ☐

Time Fasted Before Eating Today: _____

Nutritional Values:

Total Steps:

What I ate/drank:	Calories	Carbs	Fiber	Sugars	Net Carbs	Protein	Fat	Other:
Totals:								

Activity	Time	Units
Totals:		

Vitamins/ Supplements

What I took:	Amount:

Weight Change:	# Review

Sleep

Average Sleep Time: _____

What worked: _____

_____

What I can improve: _____

_____

Any changes I'd like to try next week: _____

_____

_____

_____

Mind /Spirit

What worked: _____

_____

What I can improve: _____

_____

Any changes I'd like to try next week: _____

_____

_____

_____

Social

What I enjoyed the most: _____

_____

What I can improve next week: _____

_____

_____

Ideas for other social interaction next week: _____

_____

_____

_____

♡ Gratitude / Reflections ♡

What I am grateful for as I review this week: _____

_____

_____

_____

_____

Positive reflections to carry into next week: _____

_____

_____

_____

Last Week

Food

Daily average amount of water: _____

What worked: _____

_____

What I can improve: _____

_____

How I did with calories/nutrients measured: _____

_____

How I can improve: _____

_____

_____

How I did with other diet goals: _____

_____

How I can improve: _____

_____

_____

Overall how I felt about what I consumed this week: _____

_____

What I'd like to improve next week: _____

_____

Exercise

Average Daily Steps: _____

What I enjoyed most:

What I can improve:

Vitamins/ Supplements

Any impact I noticed: _____

Any changes to try: _____

Week 5

Monday	Tuesday	Wednesday	Thursday	Friday	Saturday	Sunday
Exercise/Activity Planner						
Mind/Spirit Planner						
Social Planner						

Notes:		Bedtime Goal:	Steps Goal:	Water Goal:
		Wake-Up Goal:		

Planner

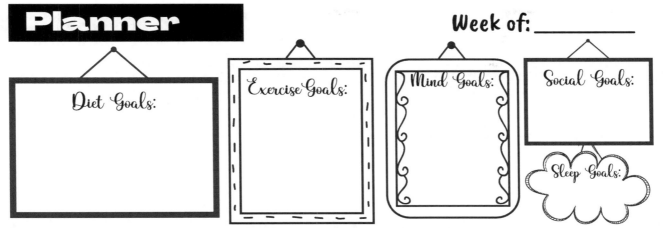

Diet Goals:

Exercise Goals:

Mind Goals:

Week of: _____

Social Goals:

Sleep Goals:

Weekly Meal Planner

Monday	Tuesday	Wednesday	Thursday	Friday	Saturday	Sunday

Weight:	# Daily

Sleep

Woke up at: _____

Total Time Slept: _____

Tonight's Bedtime: _____

Time Electronics Off: _____

Time Lights Off: _____

Room Temperature: _____

Notes: _____

_____

_____

_____

Mind / Spirit

What I did:	Time Spent:

Social

Activity:	Time Spent:

Gratitude / Reflections

Record

Food

OPEN
Eating Window Open:
_____ am / pm

CLOSED
Eating Window Closed:
_____ am / pm

Exercise

Water: ☐ ☐ ☐ ☐ ☐ ☐ ☐ Total: _____
☐ ☐ ☐ ☐ ☐ ☐ ☐ _____

Time Fasted Before Eating Today: _____

Nutritional Values:

Total Steps:

What I ate/drank:	Calories	Carbs	Fiber	Sugars	Net Carbs	Protein	Fat	Other:
Totals:								

Activity	Time	Units
Totals:		

Vitamins/ Supplements

What I took:	Amount:

Weight:	# Daily

Sleep

Woke up at: _____

Total Time Slept: _____

Tonight's Bedtime: _____

Time Electronics Off: _____

Time Lights Off: _____

Room Temperature: _____

Notes: _____

_____

_____

_____

Mind / Spirit

What I did:	Time Spent:

Social

Activity:	Time Spent:

Gratitude / Reflections

Record

Food

OPEN Eating Window Open: ___ am / pm

CLOSED Eating Window Closed: ___ am / pm

Exercise

Water: ☐☐☐☐☐☐☐ ☐☐☐☐☐☐ Total: _____

Time Fasted Before Eating Today: _____

Nutritional Values:

Total Steps:

What I ate/drank:	Calories	Carbs	Fiber	Sugars	Net Carbs	Protein	Fat	Other:
Totals:								

Activity	Time	Units
Totals:		

Vitamins/ Supplements

What I took:	Amount:

	Weight:		# Daily

Sleep

Woke up at: _____

Total Time Slept: _____

Tonight's Bedtime: _____

Time Electronics Off: _____

Time Lights Off: _____

Room Temperature: _____

Notes: _____

_____

_____

_____

Mind / Spirit

What I did:	Time Spent:

Social

Activity:	Time Spent:

Gratitude / Reflections

Record

Food

OPEN — Eating Window Open: ___ am / pm

CLOSED — Eating Window Closed: ___ am / pm

Water: ☐☐☐☐☐☐ ☐☐☐☐☐☐ Total: _____

Time Fasted Before Eating Today: _____

Nutritional Values:

What I ate/drank:	Calories	Carbs	Fiber	Sugars	Net Carbs	Protein	Fat	Other:
Totals:								

Exercise

Total Steps:

Activity	Time	Units
Totals:		

Vitamins/ Supplements

What I took:	Amount:

Daily

Sleep

Woke up at: _____

Total Time Slept: _____

Tonight's Bedtime: _____

Time Electronics Off: _____

Time Lights Off: _____

Room Temperature: _____

Notes: _____

_____

_____

_____

Mind / Spirit

What I did:	Time Spent:

Social

Activity:	Time Spent:

Gratitude / Reflections

Record

Food

OPEN Eating Window Open: am/pm

CLOSED Eating Window Closed: am/pm

Exercise

Water: ☐ ☐ ☐ ☐ ☐ ☐ Total: ☐ ☐ ☐ ☐ ☐ ☐ _____

Time Fasted Before Eating Today: _____

Nutritional Values:

Total Steps:

What I ate/drank:	Calories	Carbs	Fiber	Sugars	Net Carbs	Protein	Fat	Other:
Totals:								

Activity	Time	Units
Totals:		

Vitamins/ Supplements

What I took:	Amount:

Weight:	# Daily

Sleep

Woke up at: _____

Total Time Slept: _____

Tonight's Bedtime: _____

Time Electronics Off: _____

Time Lights Off: _____

Room Temperature: _____

Notes: _____

_____

_____

_____

Mind / Spirit

What I did:	Time Spent:

Social

Activity:	Time Spent:

Gratitude / Reflections

_____

_____

_____

_____

_____

_____

_____

_____

_____

_____

_____

_____

_____

_____

_____

_____

Record

Date: Friday / /

Food

OPEN Eating Window Open: ___ am / pm

CLOSED Eating Window Closed: ___ am / pm

Water: ☐ ☐ ☐ ☐ ☐ ☐   Total: ___
☐ ☐ ☐ ☐ ☐ ☐   ___

Time Fasted Before Eating Today: _____

Nutritional Values:

What I ate/drank:	Calories	Carbs	Fiber	Sugars	Net Carbs	Protein	Fat	Other:
Totals:								

Exercise

Total Steps:

Activity	Time	Units
Totals:		

Vitamins/ Supplements

What I took:	Amount:

Weight:	# Daily

Sleep

Woke up at: _____

Total Time Slept: _____

Tonight's Bedtime: _____

Time Electronics Off: _____

Time Lights Off: _____

Room Temperature: _____

Notes: _____

_____

_____

_____

Mind / Spirit

What I did:	Time Spent:

Social

Activity:	Time Spent:

♡ Gratitude / Reflections ♡

Record

Food

OPEN Eating Window Open: ___ am / pm

CLOSED Eating Window Closed: ___ am / pm

Water: ☐☐☐☐☐☐ Total: ☐☐☐☐☐☐ ____

Time Fasted Before Eating Today: ____

Nutritional Values:

What I ate/drank:	Calories	Carbs	Fiber	Sugars	Net Carbs	Protein	Fat	Other:
Totals:								

Exercise

Total Steps:

Activity	Time	Units
Totals:		

Vitamins/ Supplements

What I took:	Amount:

Weight:		**Daily**

Sleep

Woke up at:	
Total Time Slept:	
Tonight's Bedtime:	
Time Electronics Off:	
Time Lights Off:	
Room Temperature:	
Notes:	

Mind /Spirit

What I did:	Time Spent:

Social

Activity:	Time Spent:

Gratitude / Reflections

Record

Food

OPEN
Eating Window Open:
am / pm

CLOSED
Eating Window Closed:
am / pm

Exercise

Water: ☐☐☐☐☐☐ Total: _____
☐☐☐☐☐☐

Time Fasted Before Eating Today: _____

Nutritional Values:

Total Steps:

What I ate/drank:	Calories	Carbs	Fiber	Sugars	Net Carbs	Protein	Fat	Other:
Totals:								

Activity	Time	Units
Totals:		

Vitamins/ Supplements

What I took:	Amount:

Weight Change:	# Review

Sleep

Average Sleep Time: _____

What worked: _____

_____

What I can improve: _____

_____

_____

Any changes I'd like to try next week: _____

_____

_____

_____

Mind / Spirit

What worked: _____

_____

What I can improve: _____

_____

_____

Any changes I'd like to try next week: _____

_____

_____

_____

Social

What I enjoyed the most: _____

_____

_____

What I can improve next week: _____

_____

_____

_____

Ideas for other social interaction next week: _____

_____

_____

_____

_____

♡ Gratitude / Reflections ♡

What I am grateful for as I review this week: _____

_____

_____

_____

_____

Positive reflections to carry into next week: _____

_____

_____

_____

_____

Last Week

Food

Daily average amount of water: _____

What worked: _____

_____

What I can improve: _____

_____

How I did with calories/nutrients measured: _____

_____

How I can improve: _____

_____

_____

How I did with other diet goals: _____

How I can improve: _____

_____

_____

Overall how I felt about what I consumed this week: _____

_____

What I'd like to improve next week: _____

_____

Exercise

Average Daily Steps: _____

What I enjoyed most: _____

What I can improve: _____

Vitamins/ Supplements

Any impact I noticed: _____

Any changes to try: _____

Week 6

Monday	Tuesday	Wednesday	Thursday	Friday	Saturday	Sunday

Exercise/Activity Planner

Mind/Spirit Planner

Social Planner

Notes:	Bedtime Goal:	Steps Goal:	Water Goal:
	Wake-Up Goal:		

Planner

Diet Goals:

Exercise Goals:

Mind Goals:

Social Goals:

Sleep Goals:

Weekly Meal Planner

Monday	Tuesday	Wednesday	Thursday	Friday	Saturday	Sunday

Weight:	**Daily**

Sleep

Woke up at: _____
Total Time Slept: _____
Tonight's Bedtime: _____
Time Electronics Off: _____
Time Lights Off: _____
Room Temperature: _____
Notes: _____
_____
_____
_____

Mind /Spirit

What I did:	Time Spent:

Social

Activity:	Time Spent:

Gratitude / Reflections

Record

Date: **Monday** / /

Food

OPEN — Eating Window Open: ___ am / pm

CLOSED — Eating Window Closed: ___ am / pm

Water: ☐☐☐☐☐☐ ☐☐☐☐☐☐ Total: ____

Time Fasted Before Eating Today: ____

Nutritional Values:

What I ate/drank:	Calories	Carbs	Fiber	Sugars	Net Carbs	Protein	Fat	Other:
Totals:								

Exercise

Total Steps:

Activity	Time	Units
Totals:		

Vitamins/ Supplements

What I took:	Amount:

Weight:	# Daily

Sleep

Woke up at:	
Total Time Slept:	
Tonight's Bedtime:	
Time Electronics Off:	
Time Lights Off:	
Room Temperature:	
Notes:	

Mind / Spirit

What I did:	Time Spent:

Social

Activity:	Time Spent:

Gratitude / Reflections

Record

Food

OPEN Eating Window Open: ___ am / pm

CLOSED Eating Window Closed: ___ am / pm

Water: ☐☐☐☐☐☐ ☐☐☐☐☐☐ Total: ____

Time Fasted Before Eating Today: _____

Nutritional Values:

What I ate/drank:	Calories	Carbs	Fiber	Sugars	Net Carbs	Protein	Fat	Other:
Totals:								

Exercise

Total Steps: _____

Activity	Time	Units
Totals:		

Vitamins/ Supplements

What I took:	Amount:

Weight:		# Daily

Sleep

Woke up at: _____

Total Time Slept: _____

Tonight's Bedtime: _____

Time Electronics Off: _____

Time Lights Off: _____

Room Temperature: _____

Notes: _____

Mind / Spirit

What I did:	Time Spent:

Social

Activity:	Time Spent:

Gratitude / Reflections

Record

Date: Wednesday / /

Food

OPEN — Eating Window Open: ___ am / pm

CLOSED — Eating Window Closed: ___ am / pm

Exercise

Water: ☐☐☐☐☐☐ ☐☐☐☐☐☐ Total: _____

Time Fasted Before Eating Today: _____

Nutritional Values:

What I ate/drank:	Calories	Carbs	Fiber	Sugars	Net Carbs	Protein	Fat	Other:
Totals:								

Total Steps: 👣

Activity	Time	Units
Totals:		

Vitamins/ Supplements

What I took:	Amount:

Weight:		**Daily**

Sleep

Woke up at:	_____
Total Time Slept:	_____
Tonight's Bedtime:	_____
Time Electronics Off:	_____
Time Lights Off:	_____
Room Temperature:	_____
Notes:	_____

Mind / Spirit

What I did:	Time Spent:

Social

Activity:	Time Spent:

♡ Gratitude / Reflections ♡

Record

Food

OPEN — Eating Window Open: ___ am / pm

CLOSED — Eating Window Closed: ___ am / pm

Exercise

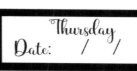

Water: ☐☐☐☐☐☐ Total: ☐☐☐☐☐☐ ____

Time Fasted Before Eating Today: _____

Nutritional Values:

Total Steps:

What I ate/drank:	Calories	Carbs	Fiber	Sugars	Net Carbs	Protein	Fat	Other:
Totals:								

Activity	Time	Units
Totals:		

Vitamins/ Supplements

What I took:	Amount:

Weight:	

Daily

Sleep

Woke up at: _____

Total Time Slept: _____

Tonight's Bedtime: _____

Time Electronics Off: _____

Time Lights Off: _____

Room Temperature: _____

Notes: _____

_____

_____

_____

Mind / Spirit

What I did:	Time Spent:

Social

Activity:	Time Spent:

♡ Gratitude / Reflections ♡

Record

Date: Friday / /

Food

OPEN — Eating Window Open: _____ am / pm

CLOSED — Eating Window Closed: _____ am / pm

Water: ☐ ☐ ☐ ☐ ☐ ☐ Total: _____
☐ ☐ ☐ ☐ ☐ ☐

Time Fasted Before Eating Today: _____

Nutritional Values:

What I ate/drank:	Calories	Carbs	Fiber	Sugars	Net Carbs	Protein	Fat	Other:
Totals:								

Exercise

Total Steps:

Activity	Time	Units
Totals:		

Vitamins/ Supplements

What I took:	Amount:

Weight:		**Daily**

Sleep

Woke up at: _____

Total Time Slept: _____

Tonight's Bedtime: _____

Time Electronics Off: _____

Time Lights Off: _____

Room Temperature: _____

Notes: _____

_____

_____

_____

Mind / Spirit

What I did:	Time Spent:

Social

Activity:	Time Spent:

Gratitude / Reflections

Record

Food

OPEN Eating Window Open: ___ am / pm

CLOSED Eating Window Closed: ___ am / pm

Exercise

Water: ☐ ☐ ☐ ☐ ☐ ☐   Total: ___
☐ ☐ ☐ ☐ ☐ ☐

Time Fasted Before Eating Today: _____

Nutritional Values:

Total Steps:

What I ate/drank:	Calories	Carbs	Fiber	Sugars	Net Carbs	Protein	Fat	Other:
Totals:								

Activity	Time	Units
Totals:		

Vitamins/ Supplements

What I took:	Amount:

Weight:		**Daily**

Sleep

Woke up at: _____

Total Time Slept: _____

Tonight's Bedtime: _____

Time Electronics Off: _____

Time Lights Off: _____

Room Temperature: _____

Notes: _____

_____

_____

_____

Mind / Spirit

What I did:	Time Spent:

Social

Activity:	Time Spent:

♡ Gratitude / Reflections ♡

Record

Food

OPEN — Eating Window Open: ___ am / pm

CLOSED — Eating Window Closed: ___ am / pm

Exercise

Water: ☐☐☐☐☐☐ Total: ___
☐☐☐☐☐☐ ___

Time Fasted Before Eating Today: _____

Nutritional Values:

Total Steps:

What I ate/drank:	Calories	Carbs	Fiber	Sugars	Net Carbs	Protein	Fat	Other:
Totals:								

Activity	Time	Units
Totals:		

Vitamins/ Supplements

What I took:	Amount:

Weight Change:	# Review

Sleep

Average Sleep Time: _____

What worked: _____

_____

What I can improve: _____

_____

Any changes I'd like to try next week: _____

_____

_____

_____

Mind /Spirit

What worked: _____

_____

What I can improve: _____

_____

Any changes I'd like to try next week: _____

_____

_____

_____

Social

What I enjoyed the most: _____

_____

_____

What I can improve next week: _____

_____

_____

_____

Ideas for other social interaction next week: _____

_____

_____

_____

_____

♡ Gratitude / Reflections ♡

What I am grateful for as I review this week: _____

_____

_____

_____

_____

Positive reflections to carry into next week: _____

_____

_____

_____

_____

Last Week

Food

Daily average amount of water: _____

What worked: _____

_____

What I can improve: _____

_____

How I did with calories/nutrients measured: _____

_____

How I can improve: _____

_____

_____

How I did with other diet goals: _____

_____

How I can improve: _____

_____

_____

Overall how I felt about what I consumed this week: _____

_____

What I'd like to improve next week: _____

_____

Exercise

Average
Daily Steps: _____

What I enjoyed most: _____

_____

_____

What I can improve: _____

_____

_____

_____

_____

Vitamins/ Supplements

Any impact I noticed: _____

_____

_____

Any changes to try: _____

_____

_____

_____

Week 7

Monday	Tuesday	Wednesday	Thursday	Friday	Saturday	Sunday

Exercise/Activity Planner

Mind/Spirit Planner

Social Planner

Notes:			Bedtime Goal:	Steps Goal:	Water Goal:
			Wake-Up Goal:		

Planner

Week of: _____

Diet Goals:

Exercise Goals:

Mind Goals:

Social Goals:

Sleep Goals:

Weekly Meal Planner

Monday	Tuesday	Wednesday	Thursday	Friday	Saturday	Sunday

Weight:

Daily

Sleep

Woke up at:	
Total Time Slept:	
Tonight's Bedtime:	
Time Electronics Off:	
Time Lights Off:	
Room Temperature:	
Notes:	

Mind / Spirit

What I did:	Time Spent:

Social

Activity:	Time Spent:

Gratitude / Reflections

Record

Food

OPEN
Eating Window Open:
_____ am / pm

CLOSED
Eating Window Closed:
_____ am / pm

Exercise

Water: ☐☐☐☐☐☐ Total: _____
☐☐☐☐☐☐

Time Fasted Before Eating Today: _____

Nutritional Values:

Total Steps:

What I ate/drank:	Calories	Carbs	Fiber	Sugars	Net Carbs	Protein	Fat	Other:
Totals:								

Activity	Time	Units
Totals:		

Vitamins/ Supplements

What I took:	Amount:

Weight:	# Daily

Sleep

Woke up at: _____

Total Time Slept: _____

Tonight's Bedtime: _____

Time Electronics Off: _____

Time Lights Off: _____

Room Temperature: _____

Notes: _____

_____

_____

_____

Mind /Spirit

What I did:	Time Spent:

Social

Activity:	Time Spent:

Gratitude / Reflections

Record

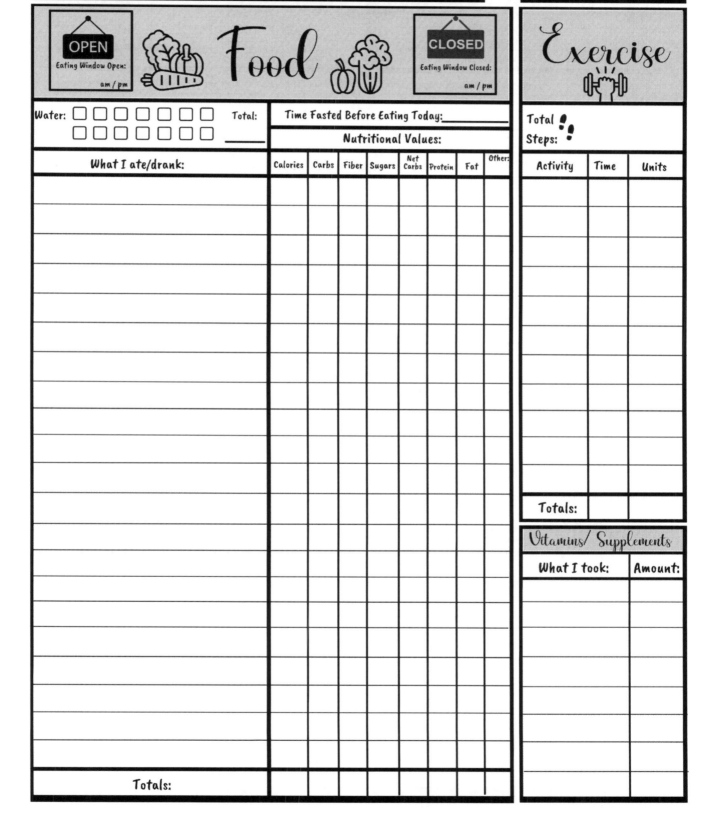

Food

OPEN — Eating Window Open: _____ am / pm

CLOSED — Eating Window Closed: _____ am / pm

Water: ☐☐☐☐☐☐ ☐☐☐☐☐☐   Total: _____

Time Fasted Before Eating Today: _____

Nutritional Values:

What I ate/drank:	Calories	Carbs	Fiber	Sugars	Net Carbs	Protein	Fat	Other:
Totals:								

Exercise

Total Steps:

Activity	Time	Units
Totals:		

Vitamins / Supplements

What I took:	Amount:

Weight:

Daily

Sleep

Woke up at:	_____
Total Time Slept:	_____
Tonight's Bedtime:	_____
Time Electronics Off:	_____
Time Lights Off:	_____
Room Temperature:	_____
Notes:	_____

Mind / Spirit

What I did:	Time Spent:

Social

Activity:	Time Spent:

Gratitude / Reflections

Record

Food

OPEN Eating Window Open: ___ am / pm

CLOSED Eating Window Closed: ___ am / pm

Exercise

Water: ☐☐☐☐☐☐ ☐☐☐☐☐☐ Total: _____

Time Fasted Before Eating Today: _____

Nutritional Values:

Total Steps:

What I ate/drank:	Calories	Carbs	Fiber	Sugars	Net Carbs	Protein	Fat	Other:
Totals:								

Activity	Time	Units
Totals:		

Vitamins/ Supplements

What I took:	Amount:

Weight:	# Daily

Sleep

Woke up at: _____

Total Time Slept: _____

Tonight's Bedtime: _____

Time Electronics Off: _____

Time Lights Off: _____

Room Temperature: _____

Notes: _____

_____

_____

_____

Mind / Spirit

What I did:	Time Spent:

Social

Activity:	Time Spent:

Gratitude / Reflections

Record

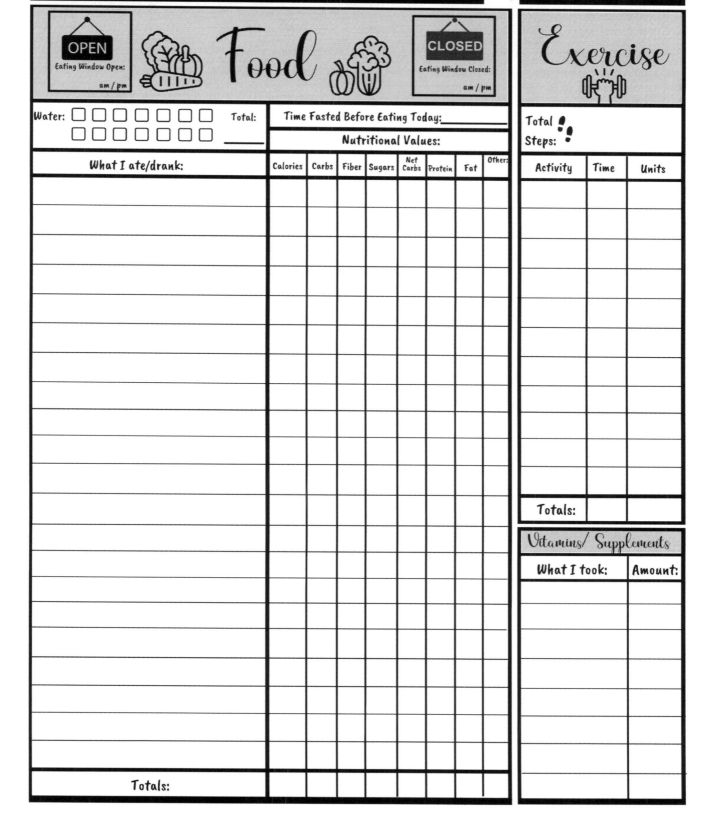

Food

OPEN Eating Window Open: ___ am / pm

CLOSED Eating Window Closed: ___ am / pm

Water: ☐ ☐ ☐ ☐ ☐ ☐ | Total:
☐ ☐ ☐ ☐ ☐ ☐ | _____

Time Fasted Before Eating Today: _____

Nutritional Values:

What I ate/drank:	Calories	Carbs	Fiber	Sugars	Net Carbs	Protein	Fat	Other:
Totals:								

Exercise

Total Steps:

Activity	Time	Units
Totals:		

Vitamins/ Supplements

What I took:	Amount:

Weight:	# Daily

Sleep

Woke up at: _____

Total Time Slept: _____

Tonight's Bedtime: _____

Time Electronics Off: _____

Time Lights Off: _____

Room Temperature: _____

Notes: _____

_____

_____

_____

Mind / Spirit

What I did:	Time Spent:

Social

Activity:	Time Spent:

Gratitude / Reflections

Record

Food

OPEN — Eating Window Open: ___ am / pm

CLOSED — Eating Window Closed: ___ am / pm

Exercise

Water: ☐ ☐ ☐ ☐ ☐ ☐ ☐ ☐ ☐ ☐ ☐ ☐   Total: _____

Time Fasted Before Eating Today: _____

Nutritional Values:

Total Steps:

What I ate/drank:	Calories	Carbs	Fiber	Sugars	Net Carbs	Protein	Fat	Other:
Totals:								

Activity	Time	Units
Totals:		

Vitamins/ Supplements

What I took:	Amount:

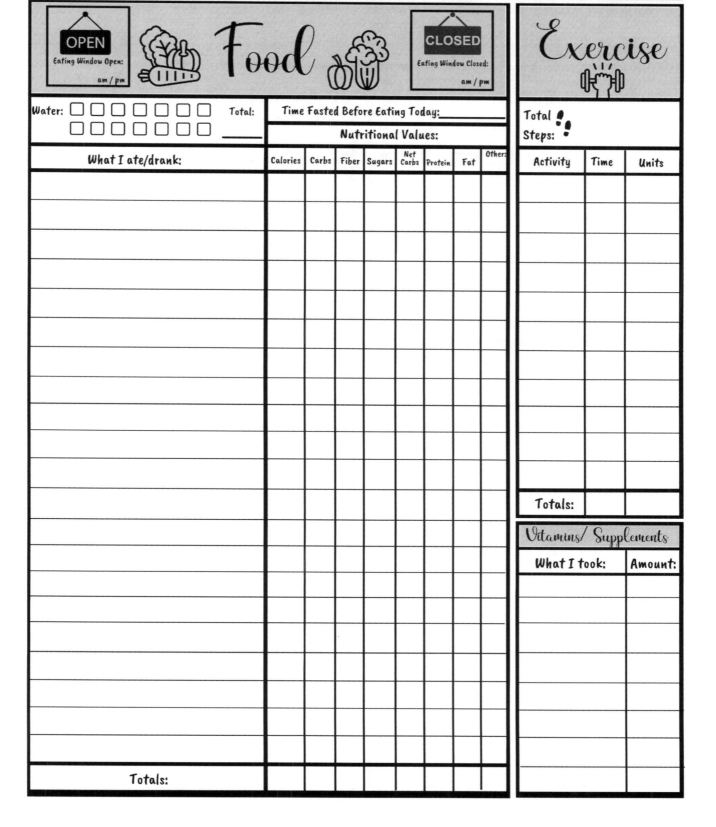

Weight:	# Daily

Sleep

Woke up at: _____

Total Time Slept: _____

Tonight's Bedtime: _____

Time Electronics Off: _____

Time Lights Off: _____

Room Temperature: _____

Notes: _____

_____

_____

_____

Mind / Spirit

What I did:	Time Spent:

Social

Activity:	Time Spent:

♡ Gratitude / Reflections ♡

Record

Food

OPEN
Eating Window Open:
am / pm

CLOSED
Eating Window Closed:
am / pm

Exercise

Water: ☐☐☐☐☐☐☐ Total:
☐☐☐☐☐☐☐ _____

Time Fasted Before Eating Today: _____

Nutritional Values:

Total Steps:

What I ate/drank:	Calories	Carbs	Fiber	Sugars	Net Carbs	Protein	Fat	Other:
Totals:								

Activity	Time	Units
Totals:		

Vitamins/ Supplements

What I took:	Amount:

Weight:

Daily

Sleep

Woke up at: _____

Total Time Slept: _____

Tonight's Bedtime: _____

Time Electronics Off: _____

Time Lights Off: _____

Room Temperature: _____

Notes: _____

_____

_____

Mind / Spirit

What I did:	Time Spent:

Social

Activity:	Time Spent:

Gratitude / Reflections

Record

Food

OPEN
Eating Window Open:
am / pm

CLOSED
Eating Window Closed:
am / pm

Exercise

Water: ☐☐☐☐☐☐ Total: ☐☐☐☐☐☐ _____

Time Fasted Before Eating Today: _____

Nutritional Values:

Total Steps:

What I ate/drank:	Calories	Carbs	Fiber	Sugars	Net Carbs	Protein	Fat	Other:
Totals:								

Activity	Time	Units
Totals:		

Vitamins/ Supplements

What I took:	Amount:

Last Week

Food

Daily average amount of water: _____

    What worked: _____

_____

    What I can improve: _____

_____

How I did with calories/nutrients measured: _____

_____

    How I can improve: _____

_____

_____

How I did with other diet goals: _____

_____

    How I can improve: _____

_____

_____

Overall how I felt about what I consumed this week: _____

_____

What I'd like to improve next week: _____

_____

_____

Exercise

Average Daily Steps: _____

What I enjoyed most: _____

_____

_____

_____

What I can improve: _____

_____

_____

_____

_____

_____

Vitamins/ Supplements

Any impact I noticed: _____

_____

_____

Any changes to try: _____

_____

_____

_____

Weight Change:	# Review

Sleep

Average Sleep Time: _____

What worked: _____

_____

What I can improve: _____

_____

Any changes I'd like to try next week: _____

_____

_____

_____

Mind /Spirit

What worked: _____

_____

What I can improve: _____

_____

Any changes I'd like to try next week:_____

_____

_____

_____

Social

What I enjoyed the most:_____

_____

_____

What I can improve next week:_____

_____

_____

Ideas for other social interaction next week:_____

_____

_____

_____

♡ Gratitude / Reflections ♡

What I am grateful for as I review this week:_____

_____

_____

_____

Positive reflections to carry into next week:_____

_____

_____

_____

_____

Week 8

Monday	Tuesday	Wednesday	Thursday	Friday	Saturday	Sunday

Exercise/Activity Planner

Monday	Tuesday	Wednesday	Thursday	Friday	Saturday	Sunday

Mind/Spirit Planner

Social Planner

Notes:				Bedtime Goal:	Steps Goal:	Water Goal:
				Wake-Up Goal:		

Planner

Diet Goals:

Exercise Goals:

Mind Goals:

Social Goals:

Sleep Goals:

Weekly Meal Planner

Monday	Tuesday	Wednesday	Thursday	Friday	Saturday	Sunday

Weight:

Sleep

Woke up at: _____

Total Time Slept: _____

Tonight's Bedtime: _____

Time Electronics Off: _____

Time Lights Off: _____

Room Temperature: _____

Notes: _____

_____

_____

_____

Mind / Spirit

What I did:	Time Spent:

Social

Activity:	Time Spent:

Gratitude / Reflections

Record

Date: Monday / /

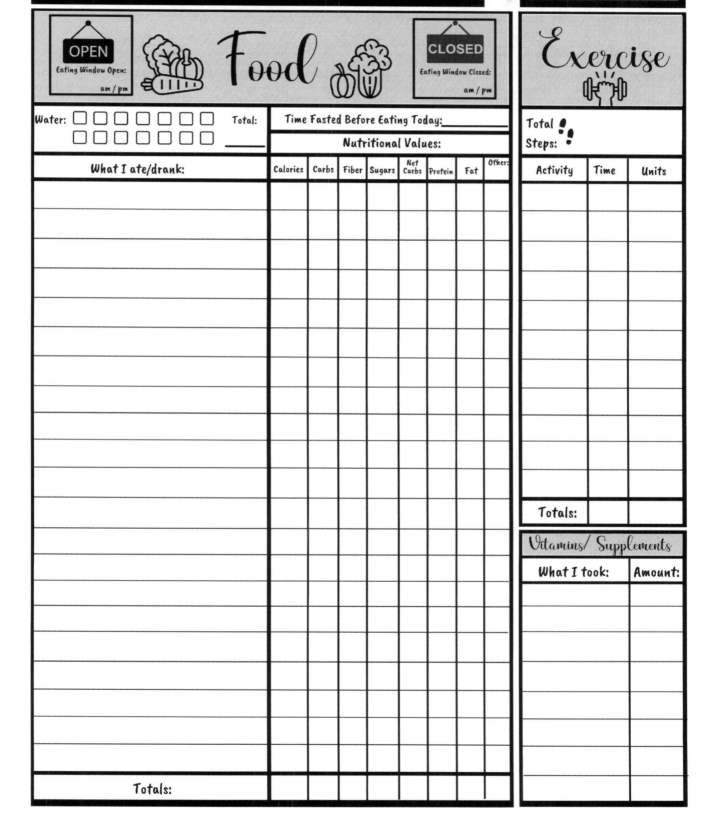

Food

OPEN Eating Window Open: ___ am / pm

CLOSED Eating Window Closed: ___ am / pm

Water: ☐☐☐☐☐☐ ☐☐☐☐☐☐ Total: ____

Time Fasted Before Eating Today: _____

Nutritional Values:

What I ate/drank:	Calories	Carbs	Fiber	Sugars	Net Carbs	Protein	Fat	Other:
Totals:								

Exercise

Total Steps:

Activity	Time	Units
Totals:		

Vitamins/ Supplements

What I took:	Amount:

Weight:	# Daily

Sleep

Woke up at: _____

Total Time Slept: _____

Tonight's Bedtime: _____

Time Electronics Off: _____

Time Lights Off: _____

Room Temperature: _____

Notes: _____

_____

_____

_____

Mind /Spirit

What I did:	Time Spent:

Social

Activity:	Time Spent:

Gratitude / Reflections

Record

Date: _Tuesday_ / /

OPEN	Food	CLOSED	Exercise
Eating Window Open: ___ am / pm		Eating Window Closed: ___ am / pm	

Water: ☐☐☐☐☐☐☐ ☐☐☐☐☐☐ Total: ___	Time Fasted Before Eating Today: _____								Total Steps:

Food

What I ate/drank:	Calories	Carbs	Fiber	Sugars	Net Carbs	Protein	Fat	Other:
Totals:								

Exercise

Activity	Time	Units
Totals:		

Vitamins/ Supplements

What I took:	Amount:

Weight:	# Daily

Sleep

Woke up at: _____

Total Time Slept: _____

Tonight's Bedtime: _____

Time Electronics Off: _____

Time Lights Off: _____

Room Temperature: _____

Notes: _____

Mind / Spirit

What I did:	Time Spent:

Social

Activity:	Time Spent:

Gratitude / Reflections

Record

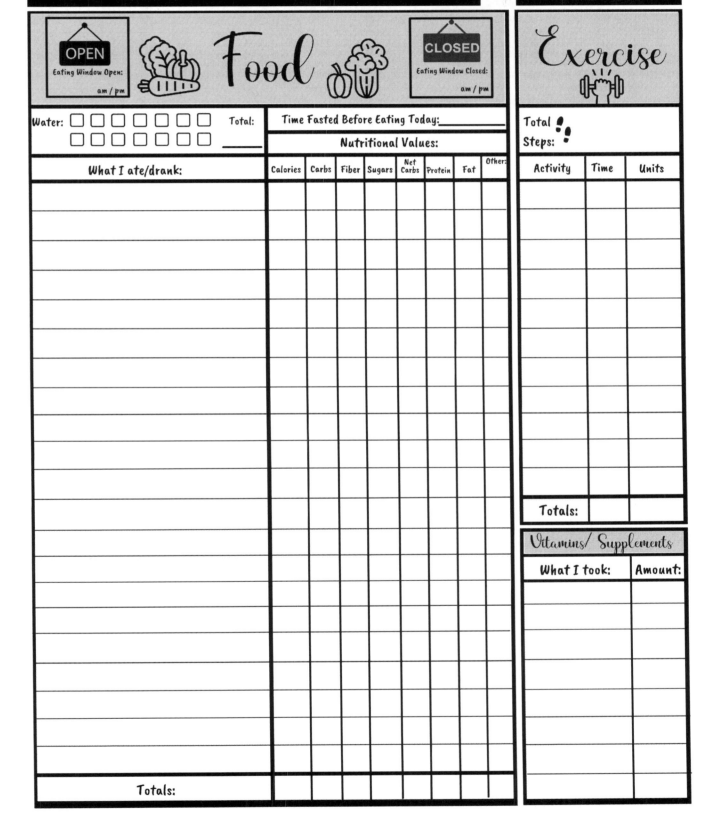

Date: Wednesday / /

Food

OPEN — Eating Window Open: ___ am / pm

CLOSED — Eating Window Closed: ___ am / pm

Exercise

Water: ▢▢▢▢▢▢ / ▢▢▢▢▢ Total: _____

Time Fasted Before Eating Today: _____

Nutritional Values:

Total Steps: _____

What I ate/drank:	Calories	Carbs	Fiber	Sugars	Net Carbs	Protein	Fat	Other:
Totals:								

Activity	Time	Units
Totals:		

Vitamins/ Supplements

What I took:	Amount:

Weight:	# Daily

Sleep

Woke up at: _____

Total Time Slept: _____

Tonight's Bedtime: _____

Time Electronics Off: _____

Time Lights Off: _____

Room Temperature: _____

Notes: _____

Mind / Spirit

What I did:	Time Spent:

Social

Activity:	Time Spent:

Gratitude / Reflections

Record

Date: Thursday __/__/__

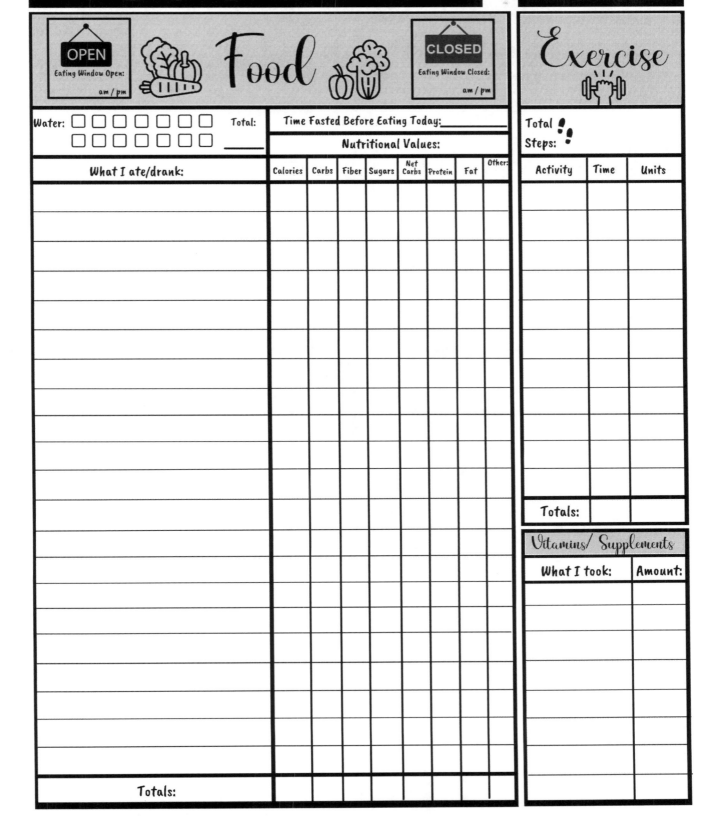

Food

OPEN — Eating Window Open: ___ am / pm

CLOSED — Eating Window Closed: ___ am / pm

Exercise

Water: ☐☐☐☐☐☐☐ ☐☐☐☐☐☐☐ Total: _____

Time Fasted Before Eating Today: _____

Nutritional Values:

Total Steps:

What I ate/drank:	Calories	Carbs	Fiber	Sugars	Net Carbs	Protein	Fat	Other:
Totals:								

Activity	Time	Units
Totals:		

Vitamins/ Supplements

What I took:	Amount:

	Weight:		**Daily**

Sleep

Woke up at: _____

Total Time Slept: _____

Tonight's Bedtime: _____

Time Electronics Off: _____

Time Lights Off: _____

Room Temperature: _____

Notes: _____

Mind / Spirit

What I did:	Time Spent:

Social

Activity:	Time Spent:

Gratitude / Reflections

Record

Food

OPEN — Eating Window Open: ___ am / pm

CLOSED — Eating Window Closed: ___ am / pm

Exercise

Water: ☐ ☐ ☐ ☐ ☐ ☐ Total: _____
☐ ☐ ☐ ☐ ☐ ☐

Time Fasted Before Eating Today: _____

Nutritional Values:

Total Steps:

What I ate/drank:	Calories	Carbs	Fiber	Sugars	Net Carbs	Protein	Fat	Other:
Totals:								

Activity	Time	Units
Totals:		

Vitamins/ Supplements

What I took:	Amount:

Weight:		# Daily

Sleep

Woke up at: _____

Total Time Slept: _____

Tonight's Bedtime: _____

Time Electronics Off: _____

Time Lights Off: _____

Room Temperature: _____

Notes: _____

Mind / Spirit

What I did:	Time Spent:

Social

Activity:	Time Spent:

Gratitude / Reflections

Record

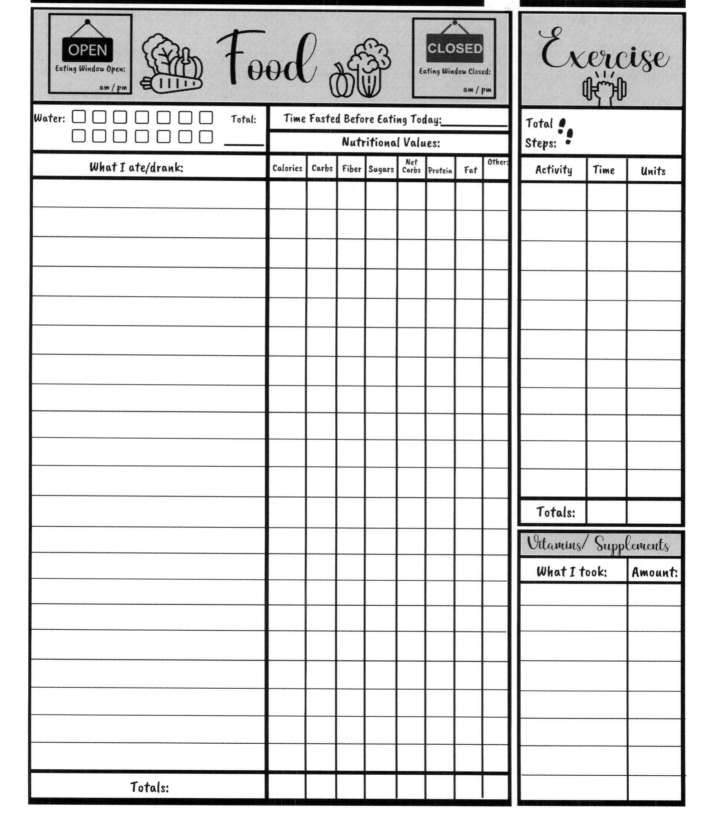

Date: Saturday / /

Food

OPEN — Eating Window Open: ___ am / pm

CLOSED — Eating Window Closed: ___ am / pm

Water: ☐☐☐☐☐☐☐ ☐☐☐☐☐☐ Total: _____

Time Fasted Before Eating Today: _____

Nutritional Values:

What I ate/drank:	Calories	Carbs	Fiber	Sugars	Net Carbs	Protein	Fat	Other
Totals:								

Exercise

Total Steps:

Activity	Time	Units
Totals:		

Vitamins/ Supplements

What I took:	Amount:

Weight:	# Daily

Sleep

Woke up at: _____

Total Time Slept: _____

Tonight's Bedtime: _____

Time Electronics Off: _____

Time Lights Off: _____

Room Temperature: _____

Notes: _____

_____

_____

_____

Mind / Spirit

What I did:	Time Spent:

Social

Activity:	Time Spent:

Gratitude / Reflections

Record

Date: Sunday / /

Food

OPEN
Eating Window Open:
am / pm

CLOSED
Eating Window Closed:
am / pm

Water: ☐ ☐ ☐ ☐ ☐ ☐ Total: ____
☐ ☐ ☐ ☐ ☐ ☐

Time Fasted Before Eating Today: _____

Nutritional Values:

What I ate/drank:	Calories	Carbs	Fiber	Sugars	Net Carbs	Protein	Fat	Other:
Totals:								

Exercise

Total Steps:

Activity	Time	Units
Totals:		

Vitamins/ Supplements

What I took:	Amount:

Weight Change:

Review

Sleep

Average Sleep Time: _____

What worked: _____

_____

What I can improve: _____

_____

_____

Any changes I'd like to try next week: _____

_____

_____

_____

Mind / Spirit

What worked: _____

_____

_____

What I can improve: _____

_____

_____

Any changes I'd like to try next week: _____

_____

_____

_____

Social

What I enjoyed the most: _____

_____

_____

What I can improve next week: _____

_____

_____

_____

Ideas for other social interaction next week: ____

_____

_____

_____

♡ Gratitude / Reflections ♡

What I am grateful for as I review this week: ____

_____

_____

_____

_____

Positive reflections to carry into next week: ____

_____

_____

_____

_____

Last Week

Food

Daily average amount of water: _____

What worked: _____

_____

What I can improve: _____

_____

How I did with calories/nutrients measured: _____

_____

_____

How I can improve: _____

_____

_____

How I did with other diet goals: _____

_____

How I can improve: _____

_____

_____

Overall how I felt about what I consumed this week: _____

_____

What I'd like to improve next week: _____

_____

_____

Exercise

Average Daily Steps: _____

What I enjoyed most: _____

_____

_____

What I can improve: _____

_____

_____

_____

_____

Vitamins/ Supplements

Any impact I noticed: _____

_____

_____

Any changes to try: _____

_____

_____

_____

Week 9

Weekly

Monday	Tuesday	Wednesday	Thursday	Friday	Saturday	Sunday
Exercise/Activity Planner						
Mind/Spirit Planner						
Social Planner						

Notes:			Bedtime Goal:	Steps Goal:	Water Goal:
			Wake-Up Goal:		

Planner

Week of: _____

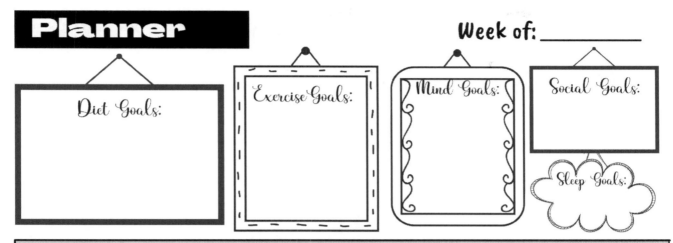

Diet Goals:

Exercise Goals:

Mind Goals:

Social Goals:

Sleep Goals:

Weekly Meal Planner

Monday	Tuesday	Wednesday	Thursday	Friday	Saturday	Sunday

Weight:	# Daily

Sleep

Woke up at: _____

Total Time Slept: _____

Tonight's Bedtime: _____

Time Electronics Off: _____

Time Lights Off: _____

Room Temperature: _____

Notes: _____

Mind /Spirit

What I did:	Time Spent:

Social

Activity:	Time Spent:

Gratitude / Reflections

Record

Date: Monday / /

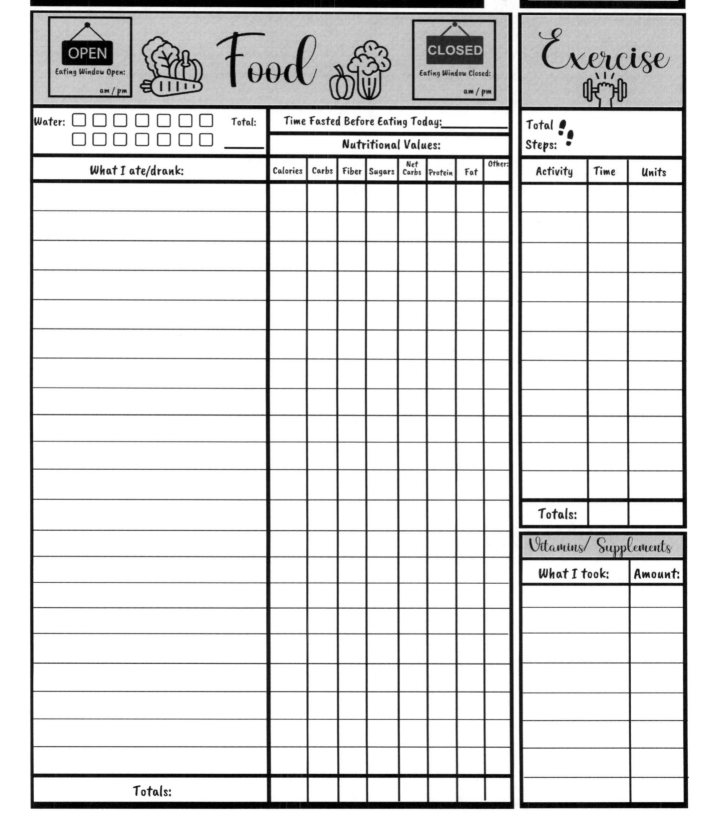

Food

OPEN — Eating Window Open: ___ am / pm

CLOSED — Eating Window Closed: ___ am / pm

Water: ☐ ☐ ☐ ☐ ☐ ☐   Total: ____
☐ ☐ ☐ ☐ ☐ ☐

Time Fasted Before Eating Today: _____

Nutritional Values:

What I ate/drank:	Calories	Carbs	Fiber	Sugars	Net Carbs	Protein	Fat	Other:
Totals:								

Exercise

Total Steps:

Activity	Time	Units
Totals:		

Vitamins/ Supplements

What I took:	Amount:

Weight:	# Daily

Sleep

Woke up at: _____

Total Time Slept: _____

Tonight's Bedtime: _____

Time Electronics Off: _____

Time Lights Off: _____

Room Temperature: _____

Notes: _____

_____

_____

_____

Mind / Spirit

What I did:	Time Spent:

Social

Activity:	Time Spent:

Gratitude / Reflections

Record

Food

OPEN Eating Window Open: am / pm

CLOSED Eating Window Closed: am / pm

Exercise

Water: ☐☐☐☐☐☐☐ ☐☐☐☐☐☐☐ Total: _____

Time Fasted Before Eating Today: _____

Nutritional Values:

Total Steps:

What I ate/drank:	Calories	Carbs	Fiber	Sugars	Net Carbs	Protein	Fat	Other:
Totals:								

Activity	Time	Units
Totals:		

Vitamins/ Supplements

What I took:	Amount:

Weight:	# Daily

Sleep

Woke up at: _____

Total Time Slept: _____

Tonight's Bedtime: _____

Time Electronics Off: _____

Time Lights Off: _____

Room Temperature: _____

Notes: _____

_____

_____

_____

Mind / Spirit

What I did:	Time Spent:

Social

Activity:	Time Spent:

Gratitude / Reflections

Record

Food

OPEN — Eating Window Open: _____ am / pm

CLOSED — Eating Window Closed: _____ am / pm

Exercise

Water: ☐ ☐ ☐ ☐ ☐ ☐ Total: _____
☐ ☐ ☐ ☐ ☐ ☐ _____

Total Steps: _____

Time Fasted Before Eating Today: _____

Nutritional Values:

What I ate/drank:	Calories	Carbs	Fiber	Sugars	Net Carbs	Protein	Fat	Other
Totals:								

Activity	Time	Units
Totals:		

Vitamins/ Supplements

What I took:	Amount:

Weight:		**Daily**

Sleep

Woke up at: _____

Total Time Slept: _____

Tonight's Bedtime: _____

Time Electronics Off: _____

Time Lights Off: _____

Room Temperature: _____

Notes: _____

_____

_____

_____

Mind / Spirit

What I did:	Time Spent:

Social

Activity:	Time Spent:

Gratitude / Reflections

Record

Food

OPEN Eating Window Open: ___ am / pm

CLOSED Eating Window Closed: ___ am / pm

Exercise

Water: ☐☐☐☐☐☐☐ Total: ☐☐☐☐☐☐☐ _____

Time Fasted Before Eating Today: _____

Nutritional Values:

Total Steps:

What I ate/drank:	Calories	Carbs	Fiber	Sugars	Net Carbs	Protein	Fat	Other:
Totals:								

Activity	Time	Units
Totals:		

Vitamins/ Supplements

What I took:	Amount:

Weight:	# Daily

Sleep

Woke up at: _____

Total Time Slept: _____

Tonight's Bedtime: _____

Time Electronics Off: _____

Time Lights Off: _____

Room Temperature: _____

Notes: _____

Mind / Spirit

What I did:	Time Spent:

Social

Activity:	Time Spent:

Gratitude / Reflections

Record

Date: Friday / /

Food

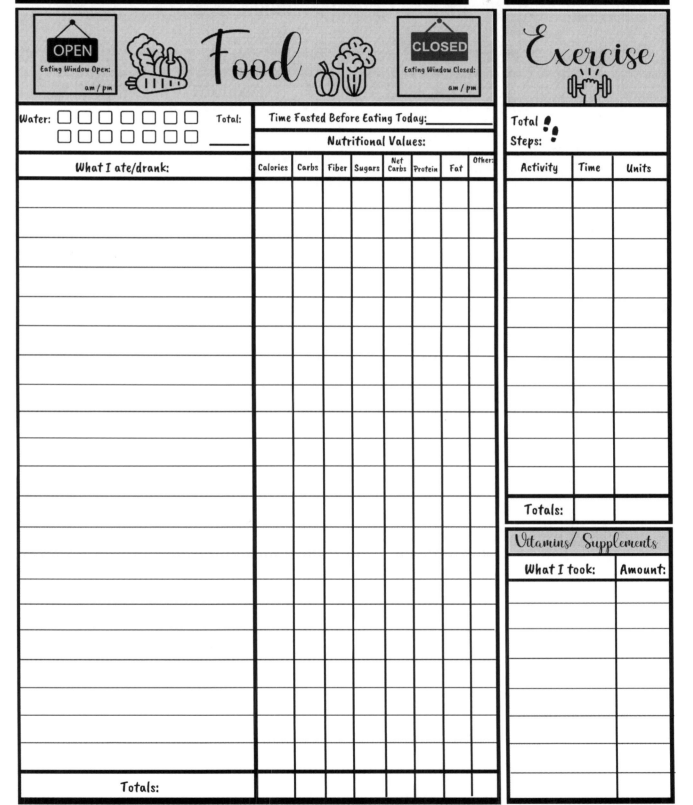

OPEN
Eating Window Open:
am / pm

CLOSED
Eating Window Closed:
am / pm

Water: ☐☐☐☐☐☐☐ Total:
☐☐☐☐☐☐ _____

Time Fasted Before Eating Today: _____

Nutritional Values:

What I ate/drank:	Calories	Carbs	Fiber	Sugars	Net Carbs	Protein	Fat	Other:
Totals:								

Exercise

Total Steps:

Activity	Time	Units
Totals:		

Vitamins/ Supplements

What I took:	Amount:

Weight:	# Daily

Sleep

Woke up at: _____

Total Time Slept: _____

Tonight's Bedtime: _____

Time Electronics Off: _____

Time Lights Off: _____

Room Temperature: _____

Notes: _____

_____

_____

_____

Mind / Spirit

What I did:	Time Spent:

Social

Activity:	Time Spent:

Gratitude / Reflections

Record

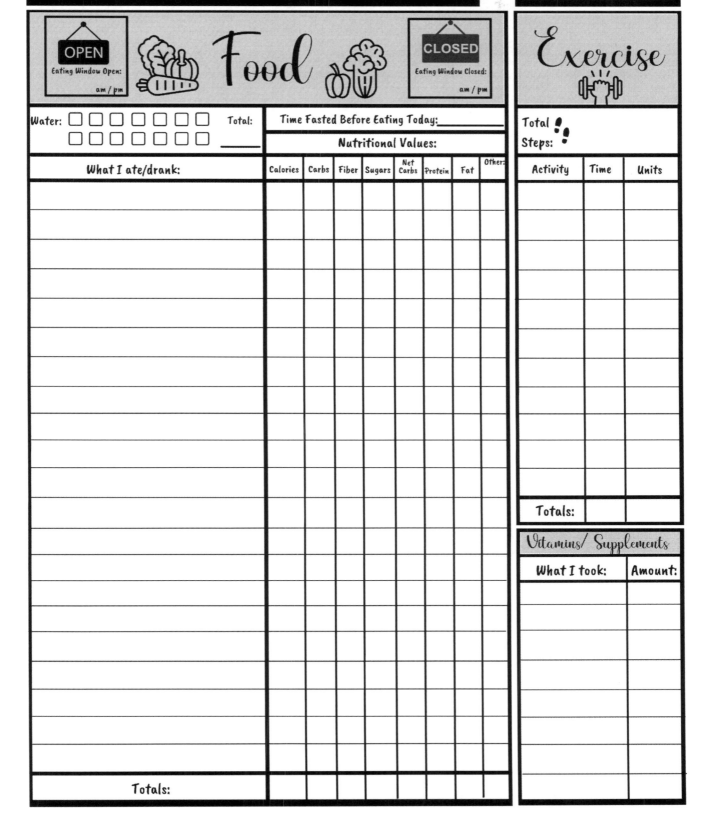

Date: Saturday / /

Food

OPEN — Eating Window Open: ___ am / pm

CLOSED — Eating Window Closed: ___ am / pm

Water: ☐☐☐☐☐☐☐ ☐☐☐☐☐☐☐   Total: _____

Time Fasted Before Eating Today: _____

Nutritional Values:

What I ate/drank:	Calories	Carbs	Fiber	Sugars	Net Carbs	Protein	Fat	Other
Totals:								

Exercise

Total Steps:

Activity	Time	Units
Totals:		

Vitamins/ Supplements

What I took:	Amount:

Weight:	# Daily

Sleep

Woke up at: _____

Total Time Slept: _____

Tonight's Bedtime: _____

Time Electronics Off: _____

Time Lights Off: _____

Room Temperature: _____

Notes: _____

_____

_____

_____

Mind /Spirit

What I did:	Time Spent:

Social

Activity:	Time Spent:

♡ Gratitude / Reflections ♡

Record

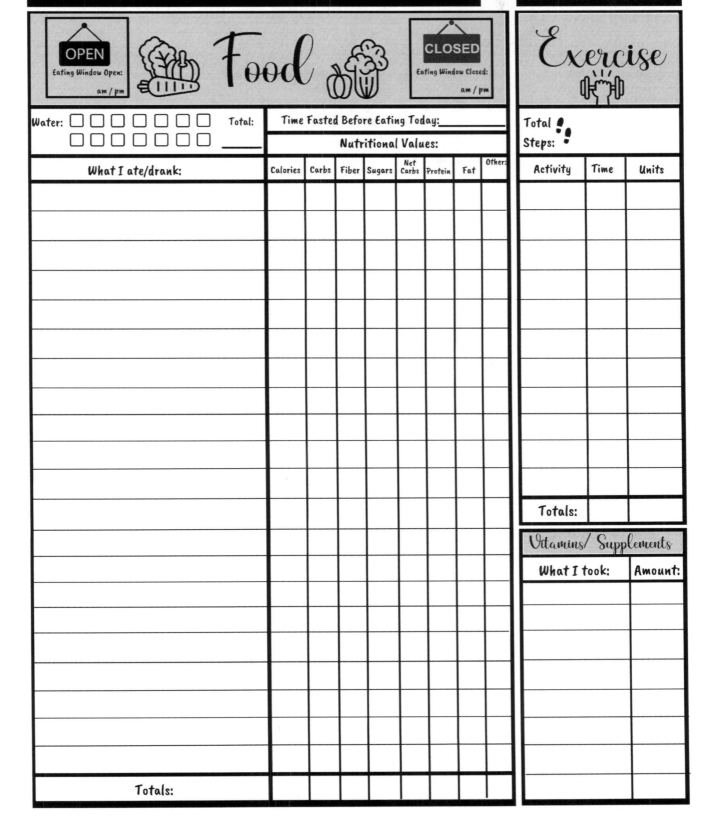

Date: Sunday / /

Food

OPEN — Eating Window Open: am / pm

CLOSED — Eating Window Closed: am / pm

Exercise

Water: ☐☐☐☐☐☐ ☐☐☐☐☐☐ Total: _____

Time Fasted Before Eating Today: _____

Nutritional Values:

Total Steps:

What I ate/drank:	Calories	Carbs	Fiber	Sugars	Net Carbs	Protein	Fat	Other:
Totals:								

Activity	Time	Units
Totals:		

Vitamins/ Supplements

What I took:	Amount:

Weight Change:	# Review

Sleep

Average Sleep Time: _____

What worked: _____

_____

What I can improve: _____

_____

Any changes I'd like to try next week: _____

_____

_____

_____

Mind /Spirit

What worked: _____

_____

What I can improve: _____

_____

Any changes I'd like to try next week:_____

_____

_____

_____

Social

What I enjoyed the most:_____

_____

_____

What I can improve next week:_____

_____

_____

_____

Ideas for other social interaction next week:_____

_____

_____

_____

♡ Gratitude / Reflections ♡

What I am grateful for as I review this week:_____

_____

_____

_____

_____

Positive reflections to carry into next week:_____

_____

_____

_____

_____

Last Week

Food

Daily average amount of water: _____

What worked: _____

_____

What I can improve: _____

_____

How I did with calories/nutrients measured: _____

_____

How I can improve: _____

_____

_____

How I did with other diet goals: _____

_____

How I can improve: _____

_____

_____

Overall how I felt about what I consumed this week: _____

_____

What I'd like to improve next week: _____

_____

_____

Exercise

Average
Daily Steps: _____

What I enjoyed most:

_____

_____

What I can improve:

_____

_____

_____

_____

_____

Vitamins/ Supplements

Any impact I noticed: _____

_____

_____

Any changes to try: _____

_____

_____

Week 10

Monday	Tuesday	Wednesday	Thursday	Friday	Saturday	Sunday
Exercise/Activity Planner						
Mind/Spirit Planner						
Social Planner						

Notes:	Bedtime Goal:	Steps Goal:	Water Goal:
	Wake-Up Goal:		

Planner

Diet Goals:

Exercise Goals:

Mind Goals:

Social Goals:

Sleep Goals:

Weekly Meal Planner

Monday	Tuesday	Wednesday	Thursday	Friday	Saturday	Sunday

Weight:	# Daily

Sleep

Woke up at: _____

Total Time Slept: _____

Tonight's Bedtime: _____

Time Electronics Off: _____

Time Lights Off: _____

Room Temperature: _____

Notes: _____

_____

_____

_____

Mind /Spirit

What I did:	Time Spent:

Social

Activity:	Time Spent:

♡ Gratitude / Reflections ♡

Record

Food

OPEN Eating Window Open: ___ am / pm

CLOSED Eating Window Closed: ___ am / pm

Exercise

Water: ☐☐☐☐☐☐ ☐☐☐☐☐☐ Total: _____

Time Fasted Before Eating Today: _____

Nutritional Values:

Total Steps:

What I ate/drank:	Calories	Carbs	Fiber	Sugars	Net Carbs	Protein	Fat	Other:
Totals:								

Activity	Time	Units
Totals:		

Vitamins/ Supplements

What I took:	Amount:

Weight:	# Daily

Sleep

Woke up at: _____

Total Time Slept: _____

Tonight's Bedtime: _____

Time Electronics Off: _____

Time Lights Off: _____

Room Temperature: _____

Notes: _____

_____

_____

Mind / Spirit

What I did:	Time Spent:

Social

Activity:	Time Spent:

Gratitude / Reflections

_____

_____

_____

_____

_____

_____

_____

_____

_____

_____

_____

_____

_____

Record

Food

OPEN — Eating Window Open: ___ am / pm

CLOSED — Eating Window Closed: ___ am / pm

Exercise

Water: ☐ ☐ ☐ ☐ ☐ ☐ Total: ___
☐ ☐ ☐ ☐ ☐ ☐

Time Fasted Before Eating Today: _____

Total Steps:

Nutritional Values:

What I ate/drank:	Calories	Carbs	Fiber	Sugars	Net Carbs	Protein	Fat	Other:
Totals:								

Activity	Time	Units
Totals:		

Vitamins / Supplements

What I took:	Amount:

Weight:	# Daily

Sleep

Woke up at: _____

Total Time Slept: _____

Tonight's Bedtime: _____

Time Electronics Off: _____

Time Lights Off: _____

Room Temperature: _____

Notes: _____

_____

_____

_____

Mind /Spirit

What I did:	Time Spent:

Social

Activity:	Time Spent:

Gratitude / Reflections

Record

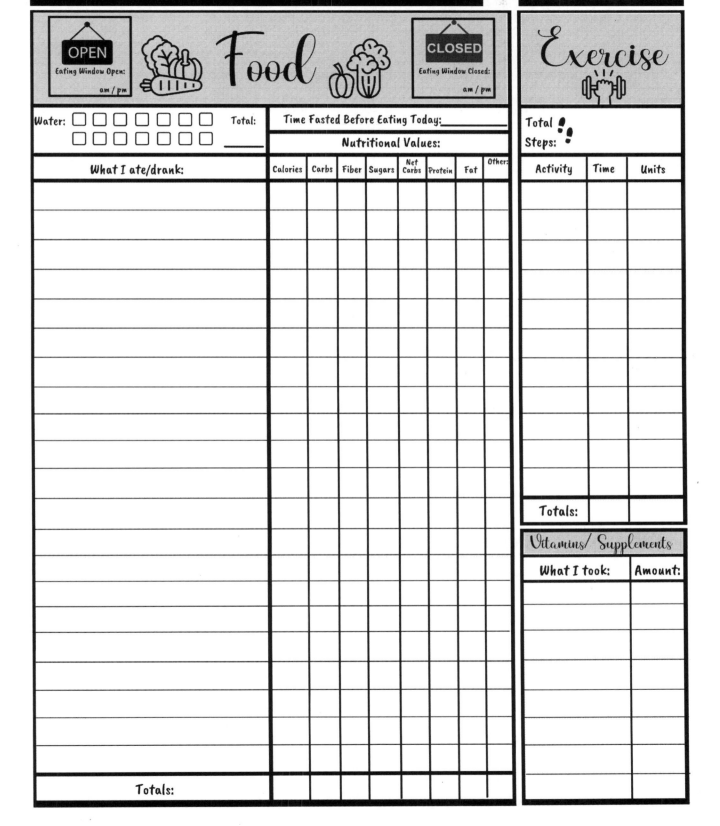

Date: Wednesday / /

Food
OPEN — Eating Window Open: ____ am / pm

CLOSED — Eating Window Closed: ____ am / pm

Exercise

Water: ☐ ☐ ☐ ☐ ☐ ☐ ☐   Total: _____
☐ ☐ ☐ ☐ ☐ ☐

Time Fasted Before Eating Today: _____

Total Steps:

Nutritional Values:

What I ate/drank:	Calories	Carbs	Fiber	Sugars	Net Carbs	Protein	Fat	Other:
Totals:								

Activity	Time	Units
Totals:		

Vitamins/ Supplements

What I took:	Amount:

Weight:	# Daily

Sleep

Woke up at: _____
Total Time Slept: _____
Tonight's Bedtime: _____
Time Electronics Off: _____
Time Lights Off: _____
Room Temperature: _____
Notes: _____
_____
_____
_____

Mind /Spirit

What I did:	Time Spent:

Social

Activity:	Time Spent:

Gratitude / Reflections

Record

Food

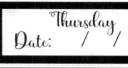

OPEN Eating Window Open: ___ am / pm

CLOSED Eating Window Closed: ___ am / pm

Exercise

Water: ☐ ☐ ☐ ☐ ☐ ☐ ☐ ☐ ☐ ☐ ☐ ☐   Total: _____

Time Fasted Before Eating Today: _____

Total Steps:

Nutritional Values:

What I ate/drank:	Calories	Carbs	Fiber	Sugars	Net Carbs	Protein	Fat	Other:
Totals:								

Activity	Time	Units
Totals:		

Vitamins/ Supplements

What I took:	Amount:

Weight:	# Daily

Sleep

Woke up at: _____

Total Time Slept: _____

Tonight's Bedtime: _____

Time Electronics Off: _____

Time Lights Off: _____

Room Temperature: _____

Notes: _____

_____

_____

_____

Mind / Spirit

What I did:	Time Spent:

Social

Activity:	Time Spent:

♡ Gratitude / Reflections ♡

_____

_____

_____

_____

_____

_____

_____

_____

_____

_____

_____

_____

_____

_____

Record

Date: Friday / /

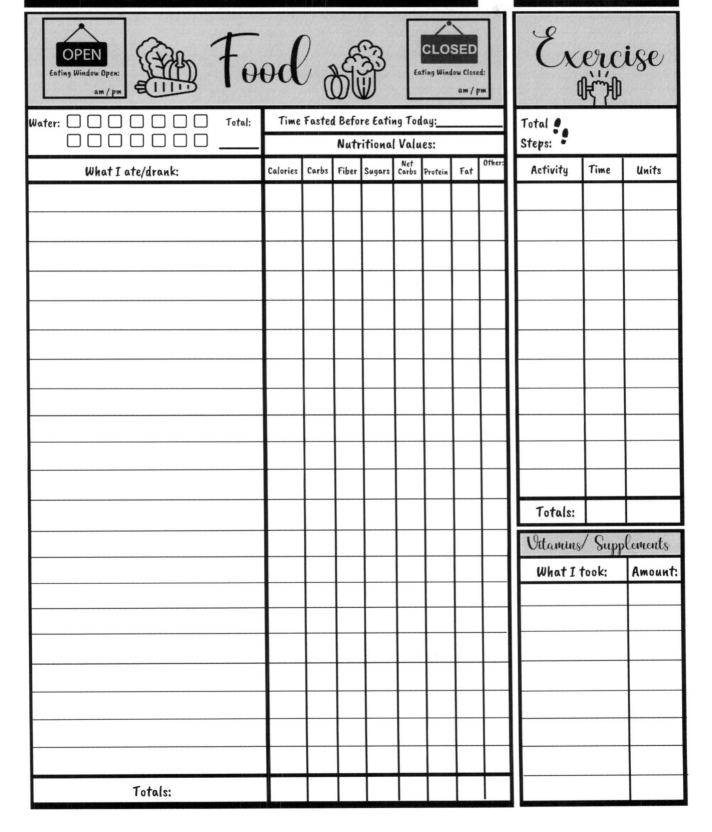

Food

OPEN — Eating Window Open: ___ am / pm

CLOSED — Eating Window Closed: ___ am / pm

Water: ☐☐☐☐☐☐ ☐☐☐☐☐☐   Total: ____

Time Fasted Before Eating Today: _____

Nutritional Values:

What I ate/drank:	Calories	Carbs	Fiber	Sugars	Net Carbs	Protein	Fat	Other:
Totals:								

Exercise

Total Steps:

Activity	Time	Units
Totals:		

Vitamins/ Supplements

What I took:	Amount:

Weight:	# Daily

Sleep

Woke up at: _____

Total Time Slept: _____

Tonight's Bedtime: _____

Time Electronics Off: _____

Time Lights Off: _____

Room Temperature: _____

Notes: _____

Mind /Spirit

What I did:	Time Spent:

Social

Activity:	Time Spent:

Gratitude / Reflections

Record

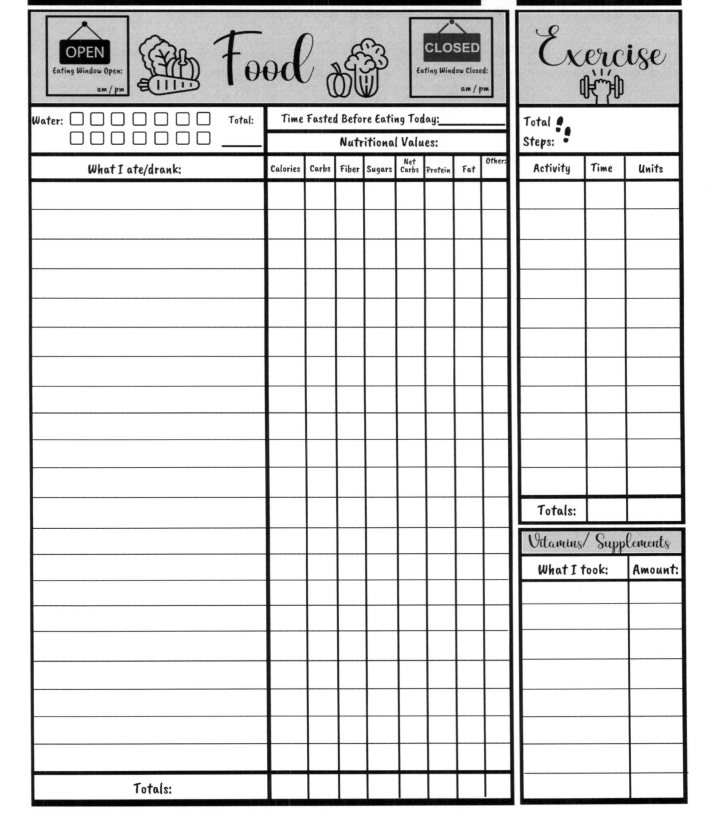

Date: Saturday / /

Food

OPEN — Eating Window Open: ___ am / pm

CLOSED — Eating Window Closed: ___ am / pm

Exercise

Water: ☐☐☐☐☐☐☐ ☐☐☐☐☐☐☐ Total: _____

Time Fasted Before Eating Today: _____

Total Steps:

What I ate/drank:	Calories	Carbs	Fiber	Sugars	Net Carbs	Protein	Fat	Other:
Totals:								

Nutritional Values:

Activity	Time	Units
Totals:		

Vitamins/ Supplements

What I took:	Amount:

Weight:		**Daily**

Sleep

Woke up at: _____

Total Time Slept: _____

Tonight's Bedtime: _____

Time Electronics Off: _____

Time Lights Off: _____

Room Temperature: _____

Notes: _____

_____

_____

_____

Mind / Spirit

What I did:	Time Spent:

Social

Activity:	Time Spent:

Gratitude / Reflections

Record

Food

OPEN Eating Window Open: am / pm

CLOSED Eating Window Closed: am / pm

Exercise

Water: ☐ ☐ ☐ ☐ ☐ ☐ Total: _____
☐ ☐ ☐ ☐ ☐ ☐

Time Fasted Before Eating Today: _____

Total Steps:

Nutritional Values:

What I ate/drank:	Calories	Carbs	Fiber	Sugars	Net Carbs	Protein	Fat	Other:
Totals:								

Activity	Time	Units
Totals:		

Vitamins/ Supplements

What I took:	Amount:

Weight Change:	# Review

Sleep

Average Sleep Time: _____

What worked: _____

_____

What I can improve: _____

_____

Any changes I'd like to try next week: _____

_____

_____

_____

Mind /Spirit

What worked: _____

_____

What I can improve: _____

_____

Any changes I'd like to try next week: _____

_____

_____

_____

Social

What I enjoyed the most: _____

_____

_____

What I can improve next week: _____

_____

_____

_____

Ideas for other social interaction next week: _____

_____

_____

_____

♡ Gratitude / Reflections ♡

What I am grateful for as I review this week: _____

_____

_____

_____

_____

_____

Positive reflections to carry into next week: _____

_____

_____

_____

Last Week

Food

Daily average amount of water: _____

What worked: _____

_____

What I can improve: _____

_____

How I did with calories/nutrients measured: _____

_____

How I can improve: _____

_____

_____

How I did with other diet goals: _____

_____

How I can improve: _____

_____

_____

Overall how I felt about what I consumed this week: _____

_____

What I'd like to improve next week: _____

_____

Exercise

Average
Daily Steps: _____

What I enjoyed most: _____

_____

_____

What I can improve: _____

_____

_____

_____

_____

Vitamins/ Supplements

Any impact I noticed: _____

_____

_____

Any changes to try: _____

_____

_____

Week 11

Monday	Tuesday	Wednesday	Thursday	Friday	Saturday	Sunday
Exercise/Activity Planner						
Mind/Spirit Planner						
Social Planner						

Notes:				Bedtime Goal:	Steps Goal:	Water Goal:
				Wake-Up Goal:		

Planner

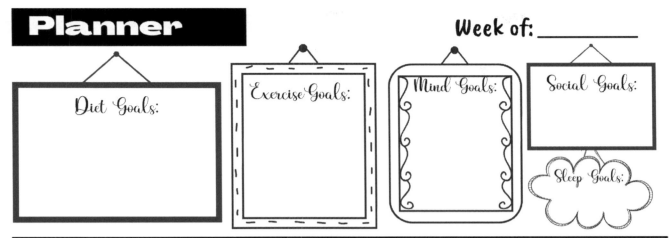

Week of: _____

Diet Goals:

Exercise Goals:

Mind Goals:

Social Goals:

Sleep Goals:

Weekly Meal Planner

Monday	Tuesday	Wednesday	Thursday	Friday	Saturday	Sunday

Weight:	**Daily**

Sleep

Woke up at: _____

Total Time Slept: _____

Tonight's Bedtime: _____

Time Electronics Off: _____

Time Lights Off: _____

Room Temperature: _____

Notes: _____

_____

_____

_____

Mind / Spirit

What I did:	Time Spent:

Social

Activity:	Time Spent:

Gratitude / Reflections

Record

Date: Monday / /

Food

OPEN
Eating Window Open:
am / pm

CLOSED
Eating Window Closed:
am / pm

Exercise

Water: ☐ ☐ ☐ ☐ ☐ ☐ | Total: ☐ ☐ ☐ ☐ ☐ ☐ _____

Time Fasted Before Eating Today: _____

Nutritional Values:

Total Steps:

What I ate/drank:	Calories	Carbs	Fiber	Sugars	Net Carbs	Protein	Fat	Other:
Totals:								

Activity	Time	Units
Totals:		

Vitamins/ Supplements

What I took:	Amount:

Weight:	# Daily

Sleep

Woke up at: _____

Total Time Slept: _____

Tonight's Bedtime: _____

Time Electronics Off: _____

Time Lights Off: _____

Room Temperature: _____

Notes: _____

_____

_____

Mind /Spirit

What I did:	Time Spent:

Social

Activity:	Time Spent:

♡ Gratitude / Reflections ♡

Record

Food

OPEN Eating Window Open: ___ am / pm

CLOSED Eating Window Closed: ___ am / pm

Exercise

Water: ☐☐☐☐☐☐ ☐☐☐☐☐☐ Total: _____

Time Fasted Before Eating Today: _____

Nutritional Values:

Total Steps:

What I ate/drank:	Calories	Carbs	Fiber	Sugars	Net Carbs	Protein	Fat	Other:
Totals:								

Activity	Time	Units
Totals:		

Vitamins/ Supplements

What I took:	Amount:

Weight:	# Daily

Sleep

Woke up at: _____

Total Time Slept: _____

Tonight's Bedtime: _____

Time Electronics Off: _____

Time Lights Off: _____

Room Temperature: _____

Notes: _____

_____

_____

_____

Mind / Spirit

What I did:	Time Spent:

Social

Activity:	Time Spent:

Gratitude / Reflections

Record

Food

OPEN Eating Window Open: ___ am / pm

CLOSED Eating Window Closed: ___ am / pm

Exercise

Water: ☐☐☐☐☐☐ ☐☐☐☐☐☐ Total: ____

Time Fasted Before Eating Today: _____

Nutritional Values:

What I ate/drank:	Calories	Carbs	Fiber	Sugars	Net Carbs	Protein	Fat	Other:
Totals:								

Total Steps:

Activity	Time	Units
Totals:		

Vitamins/ Supplements

What I took:	Amount:

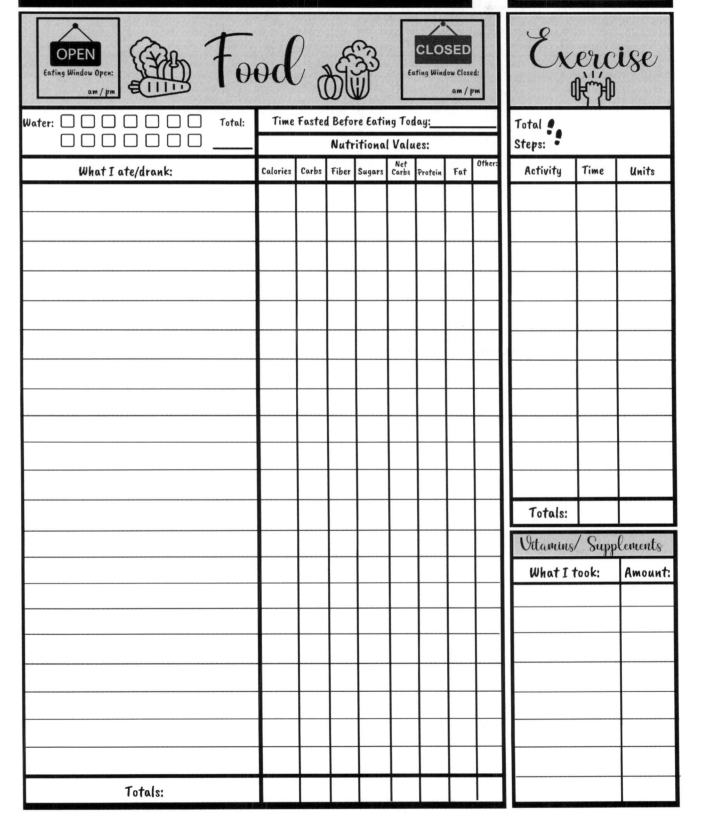

Weight:	# Daily

Sleep

Woke up at: _____

Total Time Slept: _____

Tonight's Bedtime: _____

Time Electronics Off: _____

Time Lights Off: _____

Room Temperature: _____

Notes: _____

_____

_____

_____

Mind / Spirit

What I did:	Time Spent:

Social

Activity:	Time Spent:

Gratitude / Reflections

Record

Food

OPEN Eating Window Open: ___ am / pm

CLOSED Eating Window Closed: ___ am / pm

Exercise

Water: ☐☐☐☐☐☐ ☐☐☐☐☐☐ Total: ___

Time Fasted Before Eating Today: _____

Nutritional Values:

Total Steps:

What I ate/drank:	Calories	Carbs	Fiber	Sugars	Net Carbs	Protein	Fat	Other:
Totals:								

Activity	Time	Units
Totals:		

Vitamins/ Supplements

What I took:	Amount:

Weight:	# Daily

Sleep

Woke up at: _____

Total Time Slept: _____

Tonight's Bedtime: _____

Time Electronics Off: _____

Time Lights Off: _____

Room Temperature: _____

Notes: _____

_____

_____

_____

Mind /Spirit

What I did:	Time Spent:

Social

Activity:	Time Spent:

Gratitude / Reflections

Record

Food

OPEN
Eating Window Open:
am / pm

CLOSED
Eating Window Closed:
am / pm

Exercise

Water: ☐ ☐ ☐ ☐ ☐ ☐   Total:
☐ ☐ ☐ ☐ ☐ ☐   _____

Time Fasted Before Eating Today: _____

Nutritional Values:

Total Steps:

What I ate/drank:	Calories	Carbs	Fiber	Sugars	Net Carbs	Protein	Fat	Other:
Totals:								

Activity	Time	Units
Totals:		

Vitamins/ Supplements

What I took:	Amount:

Weight:	# Daily

Sleep

Woke up at: _____

Total Time Slept: _____

Tonight's Bedtime: _____

Time Electronics Off: _____

Time Lights Off: _____

Room Temperature: _____

Notes: _____

Mind / Spirit

What I did:	Time Spent:

Social

Activity:	Time Spent:

Gratitude / Reflections

Record

Food

OPEN Eating Window Open: __ am / pm

CLOSED Eating Window Closed: __ am / pm

Exercise

Water: ☐ ☐ ☐ ☐ ☐ ☐ ☐ ☐ ☐ ☐ ☐   Total: ____

Time Fasted Before Eating Today: _____

Nutritional Values:

Total Steps: 👣

What I ate/drank:	Calories	Carbs	Fiber	Sugars	Net Carbs	Protein	Fat	Other:
Totals:								

Activity	Time	Units
Totals:		

Vitamins/ Supplements

What I took:	Amount:

Weight:	# Daily

Sleep

Woke up at: _____

Total Time Slept: _____

Tonight's Bedtime: _____

Time Electronics Off: _____

Time Lights Off: _____

Room Temperature: _____

Notes: _____

_____

_____

_____

Mind / Spirit

What I did:	Time Spent:

Social

Activity:	Time Spent:

Gratitude / Reflections

Record

Food

OPEN Eating Window Open: ___ am / pm

CLOSED Eating Window Closed: ___ am / pm

Exercise

Water: ☐☐☐☐☐☐ ☐☐☐☐☐☐ Total: ___

Time Fasted Before Eating Today: _____

Nutritional Values:

Total Steps:

What I ate/drank:	Calories	Carbs	Fiber	Sugars	Net Carbs	Protein	Fat	Other:
Totals:								

Activity	Time	Units
Totals:		

Vitamins/ Supplements

What I took:	Amount:

Weight Change:	# Review

Sleep

Average Sleep Time: _____

What worked: _____

_____

What I can improve: _____

_____

_____

Any changes I'd like to try next week: _____

_____

_____

_____

Mind /Spirit

What worked: _____

_____

_____

What I can improve: _____

_____

_____

Any changes I'd like to try next week:_____

_____

_____

_____

Social

What I enjoyed the most:_____

_____

_____

What I can improve next week: _____

_____

_____

_____

Ideas for other social interaction next week:_____

_____

_____

_____

_____

♡ Gratitude / Reflections ♡

What I am grateful for as I review this week:_____

_____

_____

_____

_____

Positive reflections to carry into next week:_____

_____

_____

_____

_____

Last Week

Food

Daily average amount of water: _____

    What worked: _____

_____

    What I can improve: _____

_____

How I did with calories/nutrients measured: _____

_____

    How I can improve: _____

_____

_____

How I did with other diet goals: _____

_____

    How I can improve: _____

_____

_____

Overall how I felt about what I consumed this week: _____

_____

What I'd like to improve next week: _____

_____

Exercise

Average
Daily Steps: _____

What I enjoyed most:

_____

_____

What I can improve:

_____

_____

_____

_____

_____

Vitamins/ Supplements

Any impact I noticed: _____

_____

_____

Any changes to try: _____

_____

_____

_____

Week 12

Monday	Tuesday	Wednesday	Thursday	Friday	Saturday	Sunday

Exercise/Activity Planner

Mind/Spirit Planner

Social Planner

Notes:			Bedtime Goal:	Steps Goal:	Water Goal:
			Wake-Up Goal:		

Planner

Diet Goals:

Exercise Goals:

Mind Goals:

Social Goals:

Sleep Goals:

Weekly Meal Planner

Monday	Tuesday	Wednesday	Thursday	Friday	Saturday	Sunday

Weight:	

Daily

Sleep

Woke up at: _____

Total Time Slept: _____

Tonight's Bedtime: _____

Time Electronics Off: _____

Time Lights Off: _____

Room Temperature: _____

Notes: _____

Mind /Spirit

What I did:	Time Spent:

Social

Activity:	Time Spent:

Gratitude / Reflections

Record

Food

OPEN
Eating Window Open:
am / pm

CLOSED
Eating Window Closed:
am / pm

Exercise

Water: ☐☐☐☐☐☐ Total: ☐☐☐☐☐☐ _____

Time Fasted Before Eating Today: _____

Nutritional Values:

Total Steps:

What I ate/drank:	Calories	Carbs	Fiber	Sugars	Net Carbs	Protein	Fat	Other:
Totals:								

Activity	Time	Units
Totals:		

Vitamins/ Supplements

What I took:	Amount:

Weight:

Sleep

Woke up at: _____

Total Time Slept: _____

Tonight's Bedtime: _____

Time Electronics Off: _____

Time Lights Off: _____

Room Temperature: _____

Notes: _____

Mind /Spirit

What I did:	Time Spent:

Social

Activity:	Time Spent:

Gratitude / Reflections

Record

Food

OPEN — Eating Window Open: am / pm

CLOSED — Eating Window Closed: am / pm

Exercise

Water: ☐ ☐ ☐ ☐ ☐ ☐   Total:
☐ ☐ ☐ ☐ ☐ ☐   _____

Time Fasted Before Eating Today: _____

Nutritional Values:

Total Steps:

What I ate/drank:	Calories	Carbs	Fiber	Sugars	Net Carbs	Protein	Fat	Other:
Totals:								

Activity	Time	Units
Totals:		

Vitamins/ Supplements

What I took:	Amount:

Weight:		**Daily**

Sleep

Woke up at: _____

Total Time Slept: _____

Tonight's Bedtime: _____

Time Electronics Off: _____

Time Lights Off: _____

Room Temperature: _____

Notes: _____

Mind /Spirit

What I did:	Time Spent:

Social

Activity:	Time Spent:

Gratitude / Reflections

Record

Food

OPEN — Eating Window Open: ___ am / pm

CLOSED — Eating Window Closed: ___ am / pm

Exercise

Water: ☐ ☐ ☐ ☐ ☐ ☐ Total: ___
☐ ☐ ☐ ☐ ☐ ☐ ___

Time Fasted Before Eating Today: _____

Total Steps:

Nutritional Values:

What I ate/drank:	Calories	Carbs	Fiber	Sugars	Net Carbs	Protein	Fat	Other:
Totals:								

Activity	Time	Units
Totals:		

Vitamins/ Supplements

What I took:	Amount:

Weight:	# Daily

Sleep

Woke up at: _____

Total Time Slept: _____

Tonight's Bedtime: _____

Time Electronics Off: _____

Time Lights Off: _____

Room Temperature: _____

Notes: _____

Mind / Spirit

What I did:	Time Spent:

Social

Activity:	Time Spent:

Gratitude / Reflections

Record

Date: _Thursday_ / /

Food

OPEN — Eating Window Open: ___ am / pm

CLOSED — Eating Window Closed: ___ am / pm

Exercise

Water: ☐☐☐☐☐☐ ☐☐☐☐☐☐ Total: ____

Time Fasted Before Eating Today: _____

Nutritional Values:

What I ate/drank:	Calories	Carbs	Fiber	Sugars	Net Carbs	Protein	Fat	Other:
Totals:								

Total Steps:

Activity	Time	Units
Totals:		

Vitamins/ Supplements

What I took:	Amount:

Weight:		**Daily**

Sleep

Woke up at:	
Total Time Slept:	
Tonight's Bedtime:	
Time Electronics Off:	
Time Lights Off:	
Room Temperature:	
Notes:	

Mind / Spirit

What I did:	Time Spent:

Social

Activity:	Time Spent:

Gratitude / Reflections

Record

Date: Friday / /

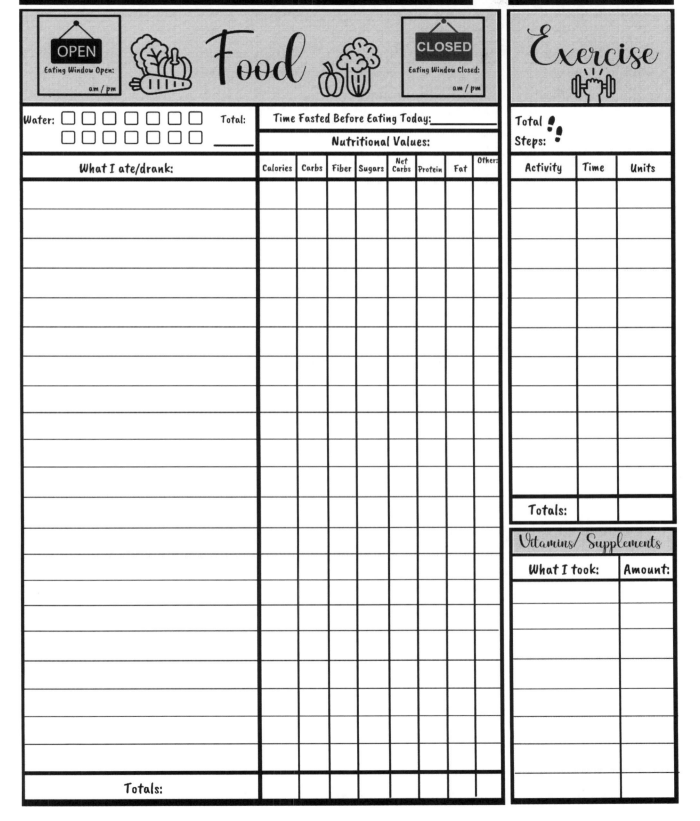

Food

OPEN — Eating Window Open: ___ am / pm

CLOSED — Eating Window Closed: ___ am / pm

Water: ☐☐☐☐☐☐ ☐☐☐☐☐☐ Total: ____

Time Fasted Before Eating Today: _____

Nutritional Values:

What I ate/drank:	Calories	Carbs	Fiber	Sugars	Net Carbs	Protein	Fat	Other:
Totals:								

Exercise

Total Steps:

Activity	Time	Units
Totals:		

Vitamins/ Supplements

What I took:	Amount:

Weight:	# Daily

Sleep

Woke up at: _____

Total Time Slept: _____

Tonight's Bedtime: _____

Time Electronics Off: _____

Time Lights Off: _____

Room Temperature: _____

Notes: _____

_____

_____

_____

Mind / Spirit

What I did:	Time Spent:

Social

Activity:	Time Spent:

Gratitude / Reflections

Record

Food

OPEN — Eating Window Open: ___ am / pm

CLOSED — Eating Window Closed: ___ am / pm

Exercise

Water: ☐ ☐ ☐ ☐ ☐ ☐ Total: ___
☐ ☐ ☐ ☐ ☐ ☐ ___

Time Fasted Before Eating Today: _____

Nutritional Values:

Total Steps:

What I ate/drank:	Calories	Carbs	Fiber	Sugars	Net Carbs	Protein	Fat	Other:
Totals:								

Activity	Time	Units
Totals:		

Vitamins/ Supplements

What I took:	Amount:

Weight: _____

Sleep

Woke up at:	_____
Total Time Slept:	_____
Tonight's Bedtime:	_____
Time Electronics Off:	_____
Time Lights Off:	_____
Room Temperature:	_____
Notes:	_____

Mind / Spirit

What I did:	Time Spent:

Social

Activity:	Time Spent:

Gratitude / Reflections

Record

Date: Sunday ___ / ___ / ___

Food

OPEN Eating Window Open: ___ am / pm

CLOSED Eating Window Closed: ___ am / pm

Water: ☐☐☐☐☐☐☐ ☐☐☐☐☐☐ Total: _____

Time Fasted Before Eating Today: _____

Nutritional Values:

What I ate/drank:	Calories	Carbs	Fiber	Sugars	Net Carbs	Protein	Fat	Other:
Totals:								

Exercise

Total Steps:

Activity	Time	Units
Totals:		

Vitamins/ Supplements

What I took:	Amount:

Weight Change:	# Review

Sleep

Average Sleep Time: _____

What worked: _____

What I can improve: _____

_____

Any changes I'd like to try next week: _____

_____

_____

_____

Mind /Spirit

What worked: _____

_____

What I can improve: _____

_____

Any changes I'd like to try next week: _____

_____

_____

_____

Social

What I enjoyed the most: _____

_____

What I can improve next week: _____

_____

_____

Ideas for other social interaction next week: _____

_____

_____

_____

♡ Gratitude / Reflections ♡

What I am grateful for as I review this week: _____

_____

_____

_____

Positive reflections to carry into next week: _____

_____

_____

_____

Last Week

Food

Daily average amount of water: _____

What worked: _____

_____

What I can improve: _____

_____

How I did with calories/nutrients measured: _____

_____

How I can improve: _____

_____

_____

How I did with other diet goals: _____

_____

How I can improve: _____

_____

_____

Overall how I felt about what I consumed this week: _____

_____

What I'd like to improve next week: _____

_____

_____

Exercise

Average Daily Steps: _____

What I enjoyed most: _____

What I can improve: _____

Vitamins/ Supplements

Any impact I noticed: _____

Any changes to try: _____

Week 13

Monday	Tuesday	Wednesday	Thursday	Friday	Saturday	Sunday

Exercise/Activity Planner

Mind/Spirit Planner

Social Planner

Notes:

Bedtime Goal:

Wake-Up Goal:

Steps Goal:

Water Goal:

Planner

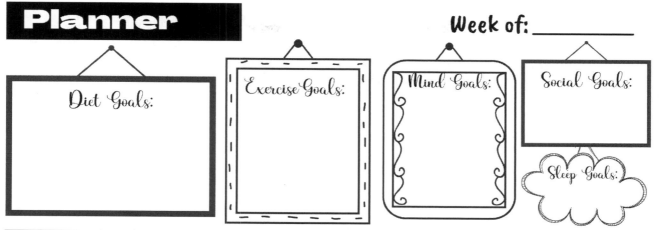

Week of: _____

Diet Goals:

Exercise Goals:

Mind Goals:

Social Goals:

Sleep Goals:

Weekly Meal Planner

Monday	Tuesday	Wednesday	Thursday	Friday	Saturday	Sunday

Weight:	# Daily

Sleep

Woke up at: _____

Total Time Slept: _____

Tonight's Bedtime: _____

Time Electronics Off: _____

Time Lights Off: _____

Room Temperature: _____

Notes: _____

_____

_____

_____

Mind /Spirit

What I did:	Time Spent:

Social

Activity:	Time Spent:

Gratitude / Reflections

Record

Date: Monday / /

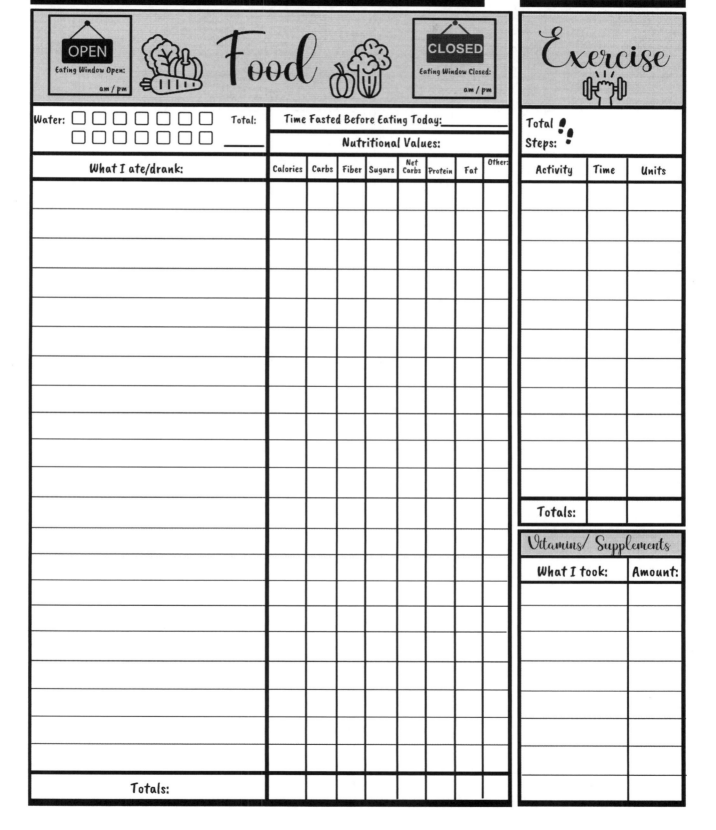

Food

OPEN — Eating Window Open: ___ am / pm

CLOSED — Eating Window Closed: ___ am / pm

Water: ☐ ☐ ☐ ☐ ☐ ☐ / ☐ ☐ ☐ ☐ ☐ ☐ Total: _____

Time Fasted Before Eating Today: _____

Nutritional Values:

What I ate/drank:	Calories	Carbs	Fiber	Sugars	Net Carbs	Protein	Fat	Other:
Totals:								

Exercise

Total Steps: _____

Activity	Time	Units
Totals:		

Vitamins/ Supplements

What I took:	Amount:

Daily

Sleep

Woke up at: _____

Total Time Slept: _____

Tonight's Bedtime: _____

Time Electronics Off: _____

Time Lights Off: _____

Room Temperature: _____

Notes: _____

Mind / Spirit

What I did:	Time Spent:

Social

Activity:	Time Spent:

Gratitude / Reflections

Weight: _____

Record

Food

OPEN — Eating Window Open: ____ am / pm

CLOSED — Eating Window Closed: ____ am / pm

Exercise

Water: ☐☐☐☐☐☐ ☐☐☐☐☐☐ Total: ____

Time Fasted Before Eating Today: _____

Nutritional Values:

Total Steps: ____

What I ate/drank:	Calories	Carbs	Fiber	Sugars	Net Carbs	Protein	Fat	Other:
Totals:								

Activity	Time	Units
Totals:		

Vitamins/ Supplements

What I took:	Amount:

	Weight:	

Daily

Sleep

Woke up at: _____

Total Time Slept: _____

Tonight's Bedtime: _____

Time Electronics Off: _____

Time Lights Off: _____

Room Temperature: _____

Notes: _____

_____

_____

Mind /Spirit

What I did:	Time Spent:

Social

Activity:	Time Spent:

Gratitude / Reflections

Record

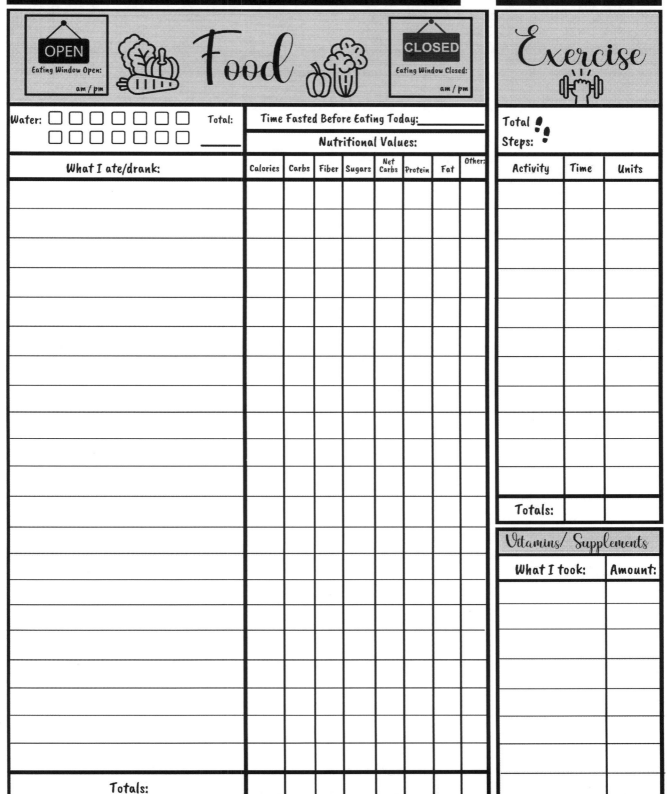

Date: Wednesday / /

Food

OPEN — Eating Window Open: ___ am / pm

CLOSED — Eating Window Closed: ___ am / pm

Exercise

Water: ☐☐☐☐☐☐ ☐☐☐☐☐☐ Total: ____

Time Fasted Before Eating Today: _____

Nutritional Values:

Total Steps:

What I ate/drank:	Calories	Carbs	Fiber	Sugars	Net Carbs	Protein	Fat	Other:
Totals:								

Activity	Time	Units
Totals:		

Vitamins/ Supplements

What I took:	Amount:

Weight:	# Daily

Sleep

Woke up at: _____

Total Time Slept: _____

Tonight's Bedtime: _____

Time Electronics Off: _____

Time Lights Off: _____

Room Temperature: _____

Notes: _____

_____

_____

_____

Mind / Spirit

What I did:	Time Spent:

Social

Activity:	Time Spent:

Gratitude / Reflections

_____

_____

_____

_____

_____

_____

_____

_____

_____

_____

_____

_____

_____

_____

_____

Record

Food

OPEN
Eating Window Open:
am / pm

CLOSED
Eating Window Closed:
am / pm

Exercise

Water: ☐ ☐ ☐ ☐ ☐ ☐ Total: _____
☐ ☐ ☐ ☐ ☐ ☐

Time Fasted Before Eating Today: _____

Total Steps:

Nutritional Values:

What I ate/drank:	Calories	Carbs	Fiber	Sugars	Net Carbs	Protein	Fat	Other:
Totals:								

Activity	Time	Units
Totals:		

Vitamins/ Supplements

What I took:	Amount:

Daily

Weight:

Sleep

Woke up at: _____

Total Time Slept: _____

Tonight's Bedtime: _____

Time Electronics Off: _____

Time Lights Off: _____

Room Temperature: _____

Notes: _____

_____

_____

_____

Mind / Spirit

What I did:	Time Spent:

Social

Activity:	Time Spent:

Gratitude / Reflections

Record

Food

OPEN
Eating Window Open:
____ am / pm

CLOSED
Eating Window Closed:
____ am / pm

Exercise

Water: ☐ ☐ ☐ ☐ ☐ ☐ ☐   Total: ____
☐ ☐ ☐ ☐ ☐ ☐

Time Fasted Before Eating Today: _____

Nutritional Values:

Total Steps:

What I ate/drank:	Calories	Carbs	Fiber	Sugars	Net Carbs	Protein	Fat	Other:
Totals:								

Activity	Time	Units
Totals:		

Vitamins/ Supplements

What I took:	Amount:

Weight:	**Daily**

Sleep

Woke up at: _____

Total Time Slept: _____

Tonight's Bedtime: _____

Time Electronics Off: _____

Time Lights Off: _____

Room Temperature: _____

Notes: _____

_____

_____

Mind / Spirit

What I did:	Time Spent:

Social

Activity:	Time Spent:

Gratitude / Reflections

Record

Date: _Saturday_ / /

Food

OPEN — Eating Window Open: ___ am / pm

CLOSED — Eating Window Closed: ___ am / pm

Exercise

Water: ☐☐☐☐☐☐ ☐☐☐☐☐☐ Total: _____

Time Fasted Before Eating Today: _____

Nutritional Values:

Total Steps: _____

What I ate/drank:	Calories	Carbs	Fiber	Sugars	Net Carbs	Protein	Fat	Other:
Totals:								

Activity	Time	Units
Totals:		

Vitamins/ Supplements

What I took:	Amount:

Weight:	# Daily

Sleep

Woke up at: _____

Total Time Slept: _____

Tonight's Bedtime: _____

Time Electronics Off: _____

Time Lights Off: _____

Room Temperature: _____

Notes: _____

_____

_____

_____

Mind / Spirit

What I did:	Time Spent:

Social

Activity:	Time Spent:

Gratitude / Reflections

_____

_____

_____

_____

_____

_____

_____

_____

_____

_____

_____

_____

_____

_____

Record

Food

OPEN
Eating Window Open:
am / pm

CLOSED
Eating Window Closed:
am / pm

Exercise

Water: ☐☐☐☐☐☐ Total: ☐☐☐☐☐☐ _____

Time Fasted Before Eating Today: _____

Nutritional Values:

Total Steps:

What I ate/drank:	Calories	Carbs	Fiber	Sugars	Net Carbs	Protein	Fat	Other:
Totals:								

Activity	Time	Units
Totals:		

Vitamins/ Supplements

What I took:	Amount:

Weight Change:

Review

Sleep

Average Sleep Time: _____

What worked: _____

_____

What I can improve: _____

_____

_____

Any changes I'd like to try next week: _____

_____

_____

_____

Mind /Spirit

What worked: _____

_____

_____

What I can improve: _____

_____

_____

Any changes I'd like to try next week:_____

_____

_____

_____

Social

What I enjoyed the most:_____

_____

_____

What I can improve next week:_____

_____

_____

_____

Ideas for other social interaction next week:_____

_____

_____

_____

♡ Gratitude / Reflections ♡

What I am grateful for as I review this week:_____

_____

_____

_____

_____

Positive reflections to carry into next week:_____

_____

_____

_____

_____

Last Week

Food

Daily average amount of water: _____

  What worked: _____
  _____

  What I can improve: _____
  _____

How I did with calories/nutrients measured: _____
_____

  How I can improve: _____
  _____
  _____

How I did with other diet goals: _____

  How I can improve: _____
  _____
  _____

Overall how I felt about what I consumed this week: _____
_____

What I'd like to improve next week: _____
_____

Exercise

Average
Daily Steps: _____

What I enjoyed most:
_____
_____
_____

What I can improve:
_____
_____
_____
_____

Vitamins/ Supplements

Any impact I noticed: _____
_____
_____

Any changes to try: _____
_____
_____
_____

Congratulations!
You did it!

13 weeks/91 days of data, evaluation, analysis, reflection, tweaking, and progressing on your journey toward total health and wellness!

Did you achieve your goals? Go back and look at your "why's" at the beginning of this book, as well as your intentions and goals. How'd you do? Is there more you'd like to do? Use this space to record your thoughts and feelings as you finish these 91 days. Make sure to also praise and reward yourself for your accomplishments!

_____

_____

_____

_____

_____

_____

_____

_____

_____

Would you like to go on for another 91 days/13 weeks?
If so, please return to Amazon to purchase another
Best Me Ever Total Wellness Planner!

Also, please consider leaving us a review on Amazon! Your
review means a lot to us and helps others make their
purchasing decisions too!
Thank you!

Made in United States
Orlando, FL
24 April 2022

17160304R00146